You Don't Have to Be Mad to Work Here

You Don't Have to Be Mad to Work Here

A PSYCHIATRIST'S LIFE

BENJI WATERHOUSE

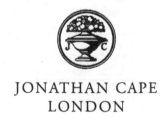

JONATHAN CAPE
LONDON

3 5 7 9 10 8 6 4

Jonathan Cape, an imprint of Vintage, is part of the Penguin
Random House group of companies whose addresses can be found at
global.penguinrandomhouse.com

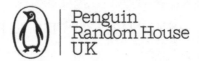

First published by Jonathan Cape in 2024

penguin.co.uk/vintage

Typeset in 11/16pt Adobe Garamond Pro by Jouve (UK), Milton Keynes
Printed and bound in Great Britain by Clays Ltd, Elcograf S.p.A.

The authorised representative in the EEA is Penguin Random House Ireland,
Morrison Chambers, 32 Nassau Street, Dublin D02 YH68

A CIP catalogue record for this book is available from the British Library

HB ISBN 9781787333178
TPB ISBN 9781787333185

Penguin Random House is committed to a sustainable future
for our business, our readers and our planet. This book is made
from Forest Stewardship Council® certified paper.

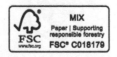

They fuck you up, your mum and dad.
They may not mean to, but they do.

Philip Larkin, 'This Be The Verse'

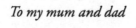

To my mum and dad

CONTENTS

PART III: Recovery

AUTHOR'S NOTE

To preserve the confidentiality of patients, colleagues and some family members, names, ages, places and identifiable details have been changed.

I have also cut most of the times when my initial response to a difficult situation was 'Shiiiiit!', but that's just to make me look cleverer.

PREFACE

I was once on an aeroplane when the call went out about a medical emergency. Being the only time since leaving medical school that this had ever actually happened, I wasn't going to miss my chance to shine.

'Let me through, I'm a doctor,' I said, elbowing my way past a gathering crowd, feeling like a hero in a film.

A pink-faced Good Samaritan with steamed-up glasses already doing CPR on a body in the aisle, looked me up and down and asked 'What *type* of doctor?'

This was clearly a more competitive gig than I'd anticipated.

I told him I was a psychiatrist.

He raised an eyebrow, turned back to the figure and muttered, 'Well I'm an emergency physician, yeah, so maybe if I manage to restart his heart, then you can ask him about his childhood.'

Admittedly in this particular case, re-establishing a pulse was a solid starting point. However, this incident reflects a widely held sentiment still prevalent today, that mental health is less important than physical health.

There has been a welcome shift in public awareness through newspapers, radio, television, podcasts, Twitter and TikTok. But the focus tends to be at the milder, more palatable end of the spectrum. Things like anxiety, depression, obsessive–compulsive disorder (OCD), autistic spectrum disorder (ASD) or the increasingly diagnosed attention-deficit hyperactivity disorder (ADHD).

Those with chronic, severe labels deemed messier, uglier or outright feared – such as schizophrenia or bipolar, personality disorders or substance-misuse disorders – receive less attention.

This book is about those people. The ones for whom some cold-water swimming and mindful colouring-in probably won't cut it. A fly-on-the-padded-wall account of my decade working in medicine's most mysterious and controversial speciality. I hope to debunk some myths about psychiatry's patients, doctors and practices (e.g. there are no padded walls).

Many people still believe that depression is caused by a 'chemical imbalance', that bipolar makes you a creative genius or that those with schizophrenia are axe-wielding murderers with 'split brains'.

Do you know the difference between a psychiatrist, a psychologist and a psychic?* Because of television, most people presume that I'm either mind-reading (that's a psychic), pitting myself against cannibalistic serial killers (that's a forensic psychiatrist), or asking wealthy, couch-strewn neurotics about their mothers (that's a psychoanalyst†). But as a general adult psychiatrist I spend my days (and often my nights) helping, or at least trying to help, predominantly those with serious mental illness.

It's often said that mental illness is no different to a broken leg. After spending six years at medical school I spent two foundation

---

* Psychiatrists are medical doctors who specialise in the diagnosis and treatment of mental illnesses and can prescribe medications (and boy do they). Psychologists help people usually with milder problems who are well enough to engage in talking therapies like CBT. And psychics mind-read and predict the future, like Mystic Meg. Fun fact: reportedly when the *Sun* newspaper's astrologer was dropped in 2015, the dismissal letter from her editor began 'As you will have no doubt foreseen . . .'

† Psychoanalysis is the classic Freudian image of a patient talking about their dreams and childhood with a cardigan-wearing analyst sitting cross-legged listening out for revealing slips of the tongue. Like when you say one thing but you mean your mother.

years as a junior doctor. During that time I treated many broken legs, mostly in A&E, and quite often in its corridors.

Back then I could see the problem either as a wonky deformity, or if I was lucky there'd be a diagnostically useful bone sticking out. When performing a physical examination I could feel the break in my hands (although the patient might prefer me not to). If I was still unsure of the diagnosis, I could perform blood tests to rule out other serious causes of bone pain like osteomyelitis. Or I could order an X-ray which would confirm the injury for me right there in black and white. Effective treatment was available too; I'd refer them to orthopaedics who would fix the break with screws, slap a plaster cast on and the patient would be pole-vaulting again in no time.

But psychiatry is different. You can't see delusional disorder, you can't feel bipolar. There is no blood test for depression. No X-rays can reveal the jagged cracks of a person's mental breakdown. You can't hold a stethoscope to someone's head and hear the voices.

Philosophically, then, where should we draw these arbitrary lines between what we call 'normal' and 'disordered', which change with time and place? Until the 1970s homosexuality was considered a mental illness which needed 'curing' with aversion therapy. And how should we treat people who venture outside our concept of normal? And is there really time to ponder this when someone who believes they're Jesus is trying to walk on water in the local swimming baths (see chapter 8)?

Another complication is that unwell patients who are disconnected from reality often lack the insight that they're unwell, so understandably won't willingly engage with treatment. At least that bloke with a backwards-facing foot suspects something is amiss.

The final potential banana skin is practical. Statistically one in four of us will experience a mental health problem at some point, and while mental illness accounts for 28% of the nation's overall disease burden, it receives just 13% of NHS funding.[1] In fact, despite increased demand for mental health support, because of deinstitutionalisation and more recently austerity, the number of psychiatric beds in England has *fallen* from 67,000 in 1988 to just 18,000 today.[2]

Consequently, acute wards run at a monthly average of over 100% with full hospitals creating extra makeshift 'beds' on ward sofas, camp beds in utility rooms, seclusion rooms and even doctors' offices. Sometimes patients are sent up to 300 miles away to the closest hospital bed. In 2019 psychiatric patients travelled the equivalent of twenty-two times around the world for 'out of area' beds[3] – can you ever imagine us making someone on crutches do that?

It is in this context – a world far away from the calm Manhattan therapy room of Woody Allen movies – that I treat my patients.

Many NHS workers cope with these challenges through gallows humour, so I hope that you won't mind that I've occasionally included some here. I think comedy can be a valuable tool for helping people to engage with difficult subjects. Also, in our battle towards parity of esteem between physical and mental health, if we'll happily laugh at the shopping list of things found up people's bodily orifices, surely we must also sometimes acknowledge the dark absurdity of the human mind. Like when someone tries to overdose on 99 paracetamols because they bought 100 but dropped one on the floor and they didn't want to get an upset tummy.

But amongst the shameful underfunding, staffing crisis, crude pharmacological treatments, and patients waiting for therapy longer than it takes the hospital Internet to load, I hope that you might find some seeds of optimism here too.

Lastly, this book is also about me and about why anyone in their right mind would choose to be a psychiatrist. I hope that it serves as a reminder that the person beneath the white coat, or in my case the elbow-patched jacket, is also human. And that the blurred lines which define what we call sanity or mental illness aren't always neatly divided by a doctor's desk.

PROLOGUE

4 a.m. The staff kettle flicks. Into a mug I add two teabags for double the hit, the boiled water, and a good glug of blue top belonging to 'Angela', knowing I'm the only one here at this time.

On the top floor I trudge along the worn institutional carpet past empty doctors' offices. Such is my status as a junior, mine is a small windowless cupboard room, otherwise known as a cupboard. I've tried to personalise it with a plant on my desk, to symbolise life. It's a cactus, though, so specifically desert life, surviving on the bare minimum, a fitting NHS metaphor. Our team secretary Cheryl, a gardening enthusiast, keeps moving it into the corridor, saying that it needs natural light. Although no one seems particularly bothered that I'm in here five days a week.

The warmth of the mug in my hands is a small comfort. I slurp some tea and fall into my chair for the first time this shift, seven hours down, six to go. I've seen eight patients already, sectioned five of them, and written precisely zero notes.

There was the man who attended A&E wondering if surgeons could remove his ears to stop the voices. The girl with anorexia nervosa whose worried parents brought her in because she refused to eat. The sleepless returning war veteran with PTSD who still couldn't lose the taste of blood in his mouth. And the usual depressing succession of common-or-garden drunks, overdoses and self-harmers.

Envious of my sleeping computer, I stir it into life. I rub my eyes then begin writing up the person I've just seen, a bloke with crystal-meth intoxication who had eaten his A&E sandwich in front of the mirror to feed his reflection.

Every day hundreds of psychiatrists attend to the troubled minds of North, South, East or West London. However at night, within my patch of the capital which covers three boroughs with a population of over 1 million, there are only five of us (because if there's one thing the mentally ill are famous for, it's long, contented sleeps).

The on-call medical team consists of one junior doctor at each of the three psychiatric hospitals, a more senior junior doctor called a registrar – that's me – advising them all over the phone while cycling around London to different A&Es to review psychiatric emergencies in person.*

Psychiatric and general hospitals are always separated, as though the mind and body are somehow disconnected, and this involves crossing the road from the 'main' hospital to the 'other' one, to use its euphemism.†

A small army of mental health nurses and social workers also help us to see the referrals which flood in from A&E,

---

* 'Junior doctor' is the confusing umbrella term used for any medic who isn't yet a consultant. All doctors do five to six years at medical school. After that, they do two more general years called F1 and F2. Then comes speciality training of varying lengths. General Practice is three more years, Psychiatry and Emergency Medicine is six, and Paediatrics is eight – probably because they waste a few years trying to convince kids that the massive needle won't hurt. Only after all of this are you no longer considered 'junior'.

† When I worked briefly in general medicine, I looked after a frail elderly woman whose devoted husband visited daily. One day he arrived to find her bed was empty and someone explained she'd 'gone upstairs'. He thanked the team for all that they'd done and went home. He was surprised a few days later to have his grieving interrupted when his wife phoned from the top floor on Geriatrics asking why he'd stopped visiting.

out-of-hour GPs, the police and hospital wards. And if we ever get *really* stuck, there's a consultant on-call at home available for telephone advice.

Only a couple of words into typing, my pager goes off, again.*

'For fuck's sake! Please . . . stop . . . calling . . . me,' I implore the little black box. It's good people can't hear the few seconds before you pick up the phone.

I punch the illuminated four digits into my desk phone and magically change personality.

'Hello this is Psychiatry, how can I help you?'

A blunt, harassed A&E matron on the other end makes her referral. 'Got one for you,' she says.

Maybe I should've been a surgeon. No one ever talks to them like that.

'Sorry, *one*?'

'A psych patient, love. You are the Psych registrar on-call aren't you?'

'Yes, I am. Can I have some more information please?'

Down the phone I hear an irritated sigh. Then the rustling of notes on a background of footsteps, squeaking trolleys and beeping machines which reassure staff their patients are still alive.

'. . . thirty-four-year-old jumped off Suicide Bridge,' she says.

Sleep-deprived, my brain wanders.

Shouldn't the council look into rebranding 'Suicide Bridge'? Something more chipper, like the 'Don't-Do-It-Viaduct' or 'Things-Will-Get-Better Overpass'?

'Dr Waterhouse?'

'Sorry yes, I'm here.' I sense the opportunity to bounce this

---

* Despite the advent of mobile phones, we still all use pagers today. If you'd like more information on the NHS's state-of-the-art communication systems, why not send them a fax?

one so I can finally make a dent in my paperwork and maybe even drink this cuppa. 'Aren't they for medics? I take it they um . . . survived?'

'Oh, you're good. Yeah they landed in some thorn bushes luckily. So just lots of superficial cuts that Plastics have sutured, and a fractured wrist that Orthopaedics have put in a pot. So we're ready for you.'

I eye my mountain of paperwork. I have one more card up my sleeve, one more opportunity to make this somebody else's problem.

'Which *side* of Suicide Bridge did they jump off?'

'What?'

'Did they jump off the north side facing the church, or the south side facing the shopping centre? It's just that that bridge divides the north and south crisis teams. We're the north one.'

'Jesus Christ,' she groans.

This isn't callous disregard for human life I tell myself, it's just the way the NHS is organised. When I'm struggling to catch my own breath, why take on cases that might come under another team's patch? Just as on a crashing plane, always apply your own oxygen mask first before helping others.

I hear the matron leaf through ambulance notes so decide to check my phone. My mum texted my family WhatsApp group eight hours earlier. Her text simply reads: 'I think Granny is dying.' None of my three younger brothers responded directly to this, not even with a sad-face emoji. It's not because we don't all love our grandmother, but because our mum Abigail is prone to drama and says this sort of thing a lot.

The next message came from my brother Gabe, several hours later, who had written 'I hope everyone is watching this?!' with a GIF of an exploding football. It's an unusual way to respond but everyone is coping with our grandmother's looming mortality

4

differently, I think, until I remember that England were playing tonight. Another cultural moment missed along with all the birthdays, weddings and Christmases that NHS employees inevitably forego.

The nurse is still audibly searching through paperwork, so hopeful, I load the BBC sports website on my phone and read about England's penalty heroics.

'OK I've found the ambulance report,' the matron announces. 'It says the patient is smelling strongly of alcohol . . . saying they wanted to die . . . best friend died yesterday . . . ah, and here it is. Discovered by a dog walker in St Martin's Church car park. So they're yours!'

Fuck fuck fuck.

I open the national online database Carenotes, which is like a Facebook for psychiatric patients.

'What's the NHS number?' I ask. I punch the numbers into the system, click search and snatch a gulp of tea while the archaic computer loads.

Then a name appears. One I know.

If my life were a film, I'd now drop my mug, the shattered ceramic bouncing off the floor in slow motion. I'd probably wail, and scream and pull at my hair too. But there's nothing cinematic about it. I've now learnt to absorb the most extreme emotions, of shock, fear or sadness with a robotic professionalism. It's easier if you don't feel too much.

'Be there shortly,' I say automatically. Then I rush off back to A&E, leaving the steaming cup of tea on my desk amongst the graveyard of other half-drunk ones.

PART I

PRODROME

noun: early signs preceding full-blown illness

1

WELCOME

'We've not printed today's timetable because the trust is £20 million in debt, so we're saving money on paper,' says Dr Laing, three years earlier, at my new-starter induction. Nightingale Hospital's clinical director is a tall, shaven-headed man in a sharp suit with the natural warmth of an ice pop. 'The news reports are true,' he continues, standing in front of a PowerPoint presentation featuring our schedule. 'The NHS is in crisis. There's a mental health epidemic and a national shortage of beds so getting one is harder than ever. Morale is low, and in real terms doctors' salaries continue to plummet. But welcome.'

For my first day in psychiatry I'm wearing the same lucky red tie my parents bought me for my medical-school interview. I somehow got in despite at one point referring to cancer as a 'growth industry' and when asked how I was with blood, I overshot my enthusiasm and said I was 'really looking forward to working with bodily fluids'.

As a junior doctor I had disregarded colleagues in other specialities who told me that psychiatrists weren't 'proper doctors'. Once, I was first at the scene of a cardiac arrest in hospital and luckily managed to resuscitate the patient.* After they were whisked away to Intensive Care my medical consultant squeezed

---

* Being the first one at a cardiac arrest is like being the first one on the dance floor at a wedding; someone's got to get it started but you'd prefer it wasn't you. And at some point it'll probably involve humming along to the Bee Gees: 'Ah, ah, ah, ah . . .'

my shoulder affectionately and said, 'Shame you're going into psych really Benji, it's a waste of a perfectly good doctor.'

I even ignored my own family. My paternal grandmother is very close to my mum but when I told her I wanted to take a slightly similar career path, not into psychology but into psychiatry, my granny shook her head and said, 'How can you have any faith in that nonsense when your mum is the way she is?'

I paid attention to none of it and now here I am, with my fellow new psychiatry trainees, probably all wondering if we've made the right choice.

Ahead of us at this induction stretch nine hours of NHS box-ticking exercises.

First we pose for photos to go on our ID badges, which a mini-printer spits out. Also on the plastic cards, the trust boasts its current CQC (Care Quality Commission) rating of 'Average', to reassure patients that they're in satisfactory hands.

A coffee break allows us newbies to mingle. I introduce myself to a plummy blonde called Beatrice. 'Benji?' she says. 'Weird name for a person. Mum used to have a golden retriever called that.' We compare war stories from our last two years working as foundation-year doctors and what brought us into medicine. I spin my polished tale of the rough diamond son of a creative child-psychologist mother and a dad who restored our family home single-handed, who grew up in rural Northumberland with just sheep for neighbours and got into medical school against all the odds. If you discount the fact that my grandpa paid for me to go to private school when I was fourteen, after I got a police caution for shoplifting (a sports bag full of Newcastle United football figurines). And that my dad went over the impossible 'practice paper' with me that the school had sent ahead of the exam. And how due to an administrative error, they hadn't actually sent me the practice paper but the exam paper itself. After sitting it, I asked my dad if we should tell the school. 'Let's not,' he said. So, we kept quiet and I got in. Still only into a low set, though, despite having seen all the questions beforehand.

We return to our seats for the final session before lunch: prevention and management of violence and aggression (PMVA) training. Otherwise known as judo.

'These are self-defence techniques you may need to use with patients,' Dr Laing tells us. 'Loose-fitting clothing is best as I once ripped my work trousers body-slamming Dr Shem. And that was before the training started.'

I bet he cracks that joke ever year.

He introduces us to Keith, a no-nonsense, middle-aged ex-policeman.

We stack away the chairs, kick off our shoes and stand in a semicircle around him like children about to go on a bouncy castle. Keith points at my tie. 'Only wear that if you want to get throttled,' he says. I remove it, resisting the temptation to tie it around my head like Rambo, and stuff it in my pocket.

'What about the ID badges?' one of the others asks.

'They're strangle-proof,' Keith says nonchalantly. 'So, if a patient grabs your NHS lanyard the release clip snaps instead of your neck.'

Keith reminds me of the over-the-top anti-drug campaigners at school who implied that one tug of a spliff would lead directly to death from a heroin overdose.

He stands in front of us and puffs out his muscular chest; his arms positioned as though he's holding a roll of carpet under each arm.

'Last year there were nearly 70,000 assaults on NHS staff and the majority of those were in a mental health setting.' Some of my new colleagues start to shift uneasily, probably wondering if that training place in radiology is still open. 'This course borrows skills from various martial arts. The techniques I'm going to teach you don't require you to be physically strong or well-built,' Keith reassures us, looking directly at me. 'Sometimes the best form of defence is attack!' he says, karate-chopping his palm for emphasis.

I wonder if that's official NHS policy?

Dr Laing raises an eyebrow at this and steps forward to try and reassert some dominance, but it's hard maintaining one's authority in socks. Especially if they're those ones that have the day of the week written on, and you're wearing Monday's on a Wednesday.

'We should also stress that violence to staff is rare,' he says. 'We're just preparing you for the worst. You should always try to avoid physically restraining a patient and injecting them with a sedative which can take up to half an hour.'

That's the problem with violence, it's *so* time-consuming.

'It's probably nicer for the patient too,' someone calls out.

'That as well,' says Dr Laing, as if that has never occurred to him. 'Violence can also cause physical and psychological harm to staff which results in time off sick* and hurts the trust financially. So always try soft skills first like offering to make them a cup of tea.'

'Although,' Keith jumps back in like a bickering divorcee, 'the most common weapon used against mental health staff is a

---

* Not going off sick is something drilled into a medic's psyche early in their training, as it gives more jobs to your already overwhelmed colleagues. When I worked briefly as a junior doctor in A&E a colleague there pushed through excruciating abdominal pain until he collapsed. On the plus side, if you are going to work through appendicitis until your gunky appendix ruptures, you could do worse than to do so fifty yards from the operating theatres. He finished off paperwork from his hospital bed.

scalding hot drink. So *never* make a ward patient a hot cup of tea.'

Dr Laing notices the startled looks on our faces as we all imagine a steaming hot Tetleys to the eyes, and steps in to reassure us. 'Such incidents are few and far between. Avoiding them is best practice. Simple things like always sitting closest to the door so you have an escape route. And using the panic alarms which will summon help immediately.'

'Presuming the batteries haven't run out,' adds Keith, ever the voice of doom.

'You can also use active listening skills,' says Dr Laing, completely ignoring Keith, 'which is where you give the impression that you're being very attentive and empathic. Let's practise demonstrating empathy,' he suggests.

'OK,' says Keith, impatient to get on to the real business of practising fighting patients. 'Can I get two volunteers?'

He points at me and a trainee wearing a headscarf called Nafisa, motioning for us to join him inside the ring. Then he makes us introduce ourselves and I resist the urge to announce WWE wrestling-style, 'In the red corner,' instead opting for a more reserved half-wave and head nod.

'OK, now one of you be verbally aggressive, don't hold back,' he commands. 'And the other try to calm them. Go!'

'Do you want to be aggressive first or should I?' Nafisa asks me with a kind smile.

'I don't mind really,' I say politely.

'OI BALDY, I'M GUNNA CUT YOUR HEAD OFF AND EAT IT!' growls Nafisa, who I think has made the executive decision to go first.

I can feel the group's eyes on me. Some are even making notes. 'Um, should we sit down and talk about that?'

'YES WE CAN SIT DOWN AND TALK ABOUT ME

CUTTING OFF YOUR BALD HEAD AND EATING IT IF YOU'D PREFER . . .'

I can't help thinking Nafisa is overdoing her performance. I allow myself a resigned, self-conscious smile.

'ARE YOU LAUGHING AT ME?!' Nafisa continues.

'No, no, I'm not. Why don't I make you a nice lukewarm cup of tea?'

'OK . . . stop,' says Dr Laing after several minutes, terminating the verbal bloodbath. 'So how did everyone feel about this scene? Let's start with what was good?'

'Well Benji seemed very calm, even when being screamed at,' someone says.

'I agree. Benji, do you have experience of being around agitated or violent people?'

Not professionally.

I shake my head.

'Well your gentle manner will be invaluable on the wards. Anything else that was good?'

A stocky trainee called Dom says it's good I didn't retaliate and punch the patient. Dr Laing nods, clearly a believer that there's no such thing as a stupid answer. The rest of us make a mental note to keep an eye on Dom.

'Now, let's talk about what could be improved?'

Beatrice, who has the quiet intensity of an all-girls' school hockey captain, looks to her notebook for inspiration. 'Well, I wouldn't say Benji's bald, more thinning . . .'

'Yeah but on the crown you can definitely see it,' Nafisa says defensively. 'He's just spiked his hair up.' The group all nod in agreement. Even Dr Laing has a subtle glance.

Worse than the embarrassment of balding is the fact that people now regularly tell me how much I look like my father John. I'll catch my reflection in shop windows and see him looking back at me. And if I've inherited his hairline, then what else?

Dr Laing interrupts my daydream. 'Now let's swap roles. This time, Benji be aggressive towards Nafisa. Again, don't hold back. Go!'

In the debrief afterwards, Beatrice says she felt that my repeatedly calling Nafisa a 'right idiot' wasn't enough. Dom suggests that I might've got more of a reaction going down the Islamophobia route. Two strikes, Dom.

Mindful of time, Keith moves us on to the main event.

'Let's first warm-up to mobilise our joints and loosen those muscles,' Keith says, lunging wildly to each side.

'I wonder if patients will hold off attacking us until we've stretched our hamstrings?' Nafisa whispers to me.

Keith demonstrates the most common types of attack – punches, kicks, grabs, holds and chokes – and how to deflect or escape them. Then we practise them in our pairs.

'Lastly some special moves to be aware of,' says Keith. 'How to remove a hand that's grabbed your hair? People have been scalped before and others dragged around like a rag doll until their neck broke. I'll spare you the gory details,' he says just one sentence too late.

He tells us it's almost impossible to get out of this one so prevention is best. He recommends short hair or hair tied up. He surveys our haircuts then points at Dr Laing and the two other entirely bald consultants. 'Excellent . . . excellent . . . excellent,' he says.

During the lunch break Nafisa and I walk past the hospital canteen's lonely-looking salad bar and join the long, motionless queue for deep-fried hot food. At some point in the day Nafisa seems to have decided that we will be friends.

'Want to play a game?' she suggests while we wait. 'It's called "psych patient or staff member". Bonus point for the difficult ones. I'll start.'

She scans the canteen then nods to a dishevelled woman sat alone eating a green apple, including the core. A giveaway stethoscope peeks out of her pocket.

'Staff member,' Nafisa says.

My turn. I move my eyes to indicate the large gentleman in front of us in the queue, in grubby clothes, with no ID badge, muttering to himself.

'Patient,' I say under my breath.

'Don't just do the easy ones,' Nafisa says.

A canteen lady wearing a hairnet leans over an empty, greasy, silver tray, and yells up the line, 'Is anyone *not* waiting for chips?' No one moves.

Suddenly, the man in front of us turns to face me and lurches his hand in my direction. I flinch and clench my fists, ready to deflect the assault as we've just practised.

'Excuse me sir,' the man says, and I realise he's just gesturing to my wristwatch. 'Have you got the time please? I've got to be back on the ward for my medicines at 2 p.m.'

In the afternoon we cover: moving and handling theory, slips, trips and falls, and in infection control how not to accidentally trigger an Ebola epidemic. I pass my competencies in handwashing training, which will now go front and centre in my CV. During a quiz at the end of the fire safety session, I learn that if a computer is in flames with live electrical wires sparking as they dance around, the best course of action is not D) Use the computer as normal.

We have a session reminding us to pay the General Medical Council and British Medical Association fees, along with

16

medical indemnity insurance which is for when doctors accidentally chop off the wrong leg. Which would be doubly concerning in psychiatry.

During a coffee break Beatrice tells us that she's worked out that new starter doctors are paid £14.09 an hour,[1] so in order to afford my London rent, professional subscriptions, the exams I must sit and pay off the £30,000 I owe the student loans company, I'm going to need to work a *lot* of hours. Which is lucky, as I will be.

At the end of the day, Dr Laing's PowerPoint reveals the individual placements we'll be on for the next year. Tomorrow morning I am to report to someone called Dr Glick.

'Finally, this is the "out of hours" rota,' Dr Laing says, changing the slide. This will dictate any social life that we attempt to have when we're not sleeping, working or revising.

'Apologies to the person working tonight, but someone's got to do it,' he says.

I'm fully expecting to have drawn the short straw but that goes to Dom. Oh well, I presume he got some shut-eye during the 'Equality and Diversity' session.

In the evening my mum calls. She never forgets an important day.

'Well love, how was it?' she asks. Her voice is sunny and calm, right in the sweet spot just one glass in.

I tell her about Dr Laing and Keith. And about some of my fellow trainees, making sure to not mention any specific female names.

'Meet anyone nice?' she adds casually. 'Nice' is code for 'potential-bearer-of-grandchildren'.

I ignore her.

'And did people like your tie?'

'Yes thanks Mum, they loved it.'

'Good. My work today just about nearly killed me,' she says.

The way my mum talks you'd think she were a firefighter who runs into burning buildings, not a psychologist who helps children with special educational needs, but everything about my mum's communication style is tinged with life-or-death levels of melodrama. Even when simply tucking me into bed as a little boy she would say: 'Benji I'd love you even if you murdered someone.' She'd say it a lot, more than simply saying, 'I love you.' So from a young age I half-expected my first kill to be just around the corner.

'Is Dad there?' I ask.

'No love, he's in the barn.'

We moved to rural Northumberland from Newcastle when I was seven, to fulfil my dad's romantic dream of building a home for his family in the remote countryside.

Moving house is considered one of the most stressful things you can do, even if you aren't swapping home comforts like central heating, running water and a roof covering the whole house for a derelict watermill that you plan to restore yourself despite not being a qualified builder, plumber, electrician or architect. But my dad had four growing boys aged seven, three, two and one to help him, so how hard could it be?

Thirty years on, long after me and my brothers have grown up and left, my dad continues trying to finish off our family home. A bit like that Japanese soldier who defended the jungle for several decades after the Second World War had finished.

'The barn' is the huge, chaotic man-shed-cum-workshop-cum-builders-yard at the end of our field. He's filled it with tools, wood of various dimensions, window frames, bags of cement, jars of screws, nails and hinges for any occasion, and random things he's found in skips. So that he's prepared if, for example, someone needs a broken piano, a cast-iron bathtub or forty primary-school chairs at short notice.

'Today he knocked down a wall which he now thinks was made entirely out of asbestos,' my mum adds.

My dad has a laissez-faire approach to health and safety. From a young age my brothers and I became handy with power tools and heavy machinery. But we never wore masks, safety goggles or hard hats. But it was OK because our dad also doubled as our family doctor. He'd worked a few years as a hospital technician in cardiology, so the human body didn't phase him. When my brother split his head open falling out of a tree or I lost four pints of blood from a gory penknife injury, our dad would manage things himself so as not to bother the professionals a fifty-minute drive away. And miraculously we are all still alive.

If my dad is often found in paint-splattered overalls, my mum likes to keep up appearances. On our family caravanning holidays she'd often be the only one who brought an ironing board with her, so that her white T-shirts weren't crumpled. My brothers and I have a memory of her, one which she denies, where she slipped getting out of the bath and fractured her dominant wrist. Even my dad realised this was a hospital job but she wouldn't let him take her until he'd helped to blow-dry her hair.

'But I called to hear about *you*,' my mum continues now.

I tell her about my induction; the health and safety stuff, the judo, and then mention the interesting afternoon session on detecting child safeguarding issues or domestic violence.

'Its tragic,' she interrupts. 'Absolutely tragic. I see it all the time in local authority work.'

My mum is an excellent child psychologist and has a whole drawer at home full of thank-you letters from grateful parents and children. She derives happiness from the positive impact that she has on children's lives. But it only gives her contentment for a while, so she's a workaholic. And it's one of her main topics of conversation, along with us boys.

She doesn't just limit her diagnoses to the kids she sees working for the council. She sometimes labels my dad as autistic or 'on the spectrum', and she jests that me and my brothers are too whenever we can't see her point of view. From our living-room sofa she once diagnosed Andy Murray with autism following one of his post-match TV interviews, but I think he was just tired.

'You're lucky you had such an idyllic childhood,' she says. I hear her swallowing, the sound of a glass being refilled.

'Yes Mum,' I say dutifully. 'Right, I'm going to do some reading before tomorrow'.

'You're just like me love. You've got my work ethic. Don't get me started on your father. He wouldn't know a career if it—'

'Mum—'

'OK, OK. Well I'm so proud of you sweetheart.'

No one is happier that I'm a doctor than my mum, who slips it into conversation wherever possible.

'My son a psychiatrist in London!' she continues. 'You're going to make such a difference to people's lives!'

2

DR GLICK

The next day at 8 a.m. I enter a concrete tower block and walk down a seemingly endless grey corridor until I reach the reinforced metal door to 'Daffodil Ward'.*

I ring the buzzer to my new workplace for the next year and study the laminated signs as I wait. One is an illustration of contraband reminding me not to bring my machete or dynamite sticks into work. Another sign respectfully implores the patients and visitors not to assault the staff. After yesterday's two-hour training session, I'd love to see them try.

Through a small pane of what looks like bulletproof glass I can see a woman with braids approaching. She unlocks the penultimate door, turns around and relocks it, then locates the correct key and unlocks the final door.

'Hi I'm Benjamin, one of the new doctors,' I explain.

'I'm Blessing, one of the nurses. Nice to meet you.' I step forward into the airlock and she begins the whole locking and unlocking and locking again rigmarole. 'You get here OK?' she asks.

'Yes thanks, I cycled. But it's good to see that staff parking is easy here if I ever get a car. There are loads of spaces!'

'That's because everyone keeps leaving. But, yeah it's good for parking,' she says, forcing a smile.

---

* Modern psychiatric wards are often named after cheerful things: local heroes, precious gems or flowers. One hospital I heard about even used Disney characters, presumably to distance themselves from the hellish associations of the asylums: the chains, rats and stark-raving madness. Much better to name the wards after normal things like a woman whose mirror can talk or a bloke who thinks his carpet can fly.

After Blessing locks the final door she reattaches the jangling keys to her belt and I follow her down a corridor, the peeling walls painted celery-green. On either side we pass what look like patient bedrooms. A healthcare assistant diligently peers in through the portholes in the bedroom doors, at the bodies still in bed.

'Obs,' says Blessing, gesturing. 'Basically suicide watch.'

I'll learn that it's not easy to kill yourself on a psychiatric ward. Belts and shoelaces are confiscated and there are no door handles to hang ligatures from anyway. Shaving with razor blades is supervised and the cutlery is counted after each meal. On top of this, patients are monitored day and night. Every time the man looks inside and sees a moving patient, he squiggles a signature on a clipboard to indicate that they've been checked, just as cleaners do in service-station toilets.

Next, Blessing and I come to a large recreational room where some early birds are already on sofas hunched around a television encased within a Perspex box. The largest patient holds the remote control and loud music blasts out.

'So this is the living area where patients can do activities like watching TV and . . . yeah, so that's the rec room,' Blessing says. 'We're an eighteen-bed mixed-admission ward. Patients come here in the usual ways. Dr Glick has the shortest length of stay in the hospital. She likes to get them out or moved on to a treatment ward within seventy-two hours.'

'Like a drive-thru,' I say.

Blessing looks at me, narrowing her eyes. 'Oh, you're one of those funny ones. Aren't we lucky.' She points me to the staff office: large panes forming a giant fish tank in the middle of the living space so patients can be observed at all times.

'Wait in there for the morning meeting. Dr Glick will be here soon. I'll join when I've finished doing morning meds.'

I head to the glass rectangle and knock and knock on the door until my knuckles hurt. The staff inside dressed in casual clothes, tapping on their keyboards, show an impressive commitment to pretending that they can't hear me. I eventually press my ID badge to the glass like a cop in a film. A well-built nurse in jeans and a T-shirt jumps up and opens the door.

'Hi I'm Benjamin, the new doctor.'

'Hello Doctor, I'm Omar. I'm so sorry I thought you were a *patient*.'

As I wait inside, staff try to focus on their endless administrative tasks as patients incessantly bang on the glass with various requests. 'Can I go on home leave?', 'Can I have a second breakfast?', 'Why are the doctors injecting me with medicine that's turning me into a frog?'

Just before 9 a.m. a woman wearing all black enters. She has hair tied up into a bun that looks as tight as her perfectly straight lips. And her shoes are so shiny I can see my own tired face in them. 'Are you Ben?' she asks.

'Benjamin, yes. Or Benji,' I say smiling.

For some reason I've always just disliked the name Ben. At least now I can establish right from the beginning of my psychiatric career that I am definitely not a Ben.

'Ben I've been waiting for you in my office,' she says. 'Get here earlier next time.'

She hasn't actually introduced herself so I study her dangling NHS lanyard. Yes, 'Dr Iva Glick', my supervisor and mentor. Who doesn't even smile for their hospital badge photo?

'Let's begin shall we? Morning Blessing,' she says as Blessing enters with the patients' medication charts. 'Oh, and we're graced with a bed manager today. Hello Brian.'

A pasty man in rectangular tortoiseshell glasses enters holding a notebook and, with a biro hanging from his lips, perches on a free section of desk.

Omar stands by the whiteboard with the least-empty marker pen. 'Good morning everyone. Overnight we had six new admissions.'

'*Six?*' everyone murmurs.

'Yeah, I don't know what was going on. Wasn't even a full moon. First up in Bed 1, we have Paige Brown.'

'How the hell did she get in?' demands Brian.

'The doctor on-call last night must've admitted her.'

'Was the warning in red capitals on her profile saying "DO NOT ADMIT AS HOSPITAL ADMISSIONS DON'T WORK" not clear enough for them?' says Brian.

'Don't forget it was Black Wednesday yesterday,' says Dr Glick.*

Blessing, who is sitting by a computer, says, 'It was a . . . Dr Dominic Bowen?'

Dr Glick wrinkles her nose. 'No, I don't know them. Sounds like a new one. I'll have a word.'

I nervously join in smiling with everyone else at this naive error without really understanding what Dom has done wrong.

Dr Glick turns to me and thrusts some paper notes in my hand. 'Right Ben. In the spirit of setting a thief to catch a thief, help us to understand why your colleague felt Paige Brown needed admitting so urgently.'

Those on office chairs swivel to look at me as I scour the pages. I scan the scrawled notes and ticked boxes until I get to his 'impression' at the bottom.

'Um, well it's quite straightforward really,' I say, confident this is an open and closed case. 'Miss Brown needed admitting urgently because she said she was going to kill herself.'

---

* Black Wednesday is the day when all junior doctors change jobs and there's a statistically significant rise in mortality rates. Not to be confused with Black Friday, which is the day when people risk their lives to get the best bargains. But at least some of them almost get their hands on a half-price telly.

At this, the team erupts with laughter.

'And my name's Santa Claus,' says Brian. 'Trust us to get the best trainees, eh Dr Glick?'

'Lesson one, Ben,' says Dr Glick. 'Do you know how much an NHS hospital bed costs? £400 per night. That's more expensive than the Ritz.'

'Although I hear they do a better breakfast,' says Brian. He's still sucking on his biro and I briefly daydream about him choking on it. 'It's all just personality disorder Ben,' he continues. 'She's a "frequent flyer" and a notorious bed-blocker, according to the notes, although I haven't had the pleasure.'* He turns to Dr Glick. 'I trust you can have her out today?'

'I'll try my best,' she says.

Brian turns to me. 'Ben, you're lucky to have Dr Glick as a mentor. She's one of the best.'

I think Dr Glick smiles, but it's hard to tell.

Brian crosses through Paige's name in his notebook. 'OK who's next?'

'In Bed 4 we have Terry Cole.'

'Terry Cole,' everyone groans. 'How the hell did he get in?'

After the meeting Dr Glick pushes some paper into my hand. 'Right Ben, I'll talk, you write,' she instructs me and I dutifully follow her into Room 1.

Paige Brown lies in front of us in bed. I'm struck by how young she seems, with a ponytail of box-dyed peroxide hair but

---

* 'Frequent flyer' I will learn is the pejorative term for those who often attend A&E. Sometimes also known as 'drug seekers', 'borderlines' or 'time-wasters'. Unlike most frequent flyers they rarely receive special treatment and are about as welcome as a screaming baby on an EasyJet flight. Some electronic systems in America even have an aeroplane logo by such patients' names to help identify them.

with sea-blue eyes that look as though they've lived through several lifetimes. Yesterday she'd been found unconscious in the street with a needle still hanging out of her arm, and with pinpoint pupils, she was treated for a suspected heroin overdose. On coming round in A&E a nurse asked if she'd like a cuppa and she said she'd rather jump out of her bedroom window, hence the psychiatry referral. Dom's job the previous night was to discern if Paige was genuinely suicidal or if she just really hated tea. He thought the former, but the rest of the team clearly think otherwise.

Dr Glick's intense gaze falls on our patient. 'Hello Paige, I'm Dr Glick the consultant psychiatrist. I know you discussed things last night with the on-call doctor, but we'll need to go through everything again. So, I gather you want to kill yourself?'

'Yeah I've had enough of it.'

'Enough of . . . ?'

'Life. My life. Every day is just pain.'

Dr Glick remains fixed to the spot, unmovable.

'That sounds exhausting,' I reflect, keen to impress Dr Glick with the communication skills that I learnt at medical school. 'Would you tell us a bit more about that?' Dr Glick's eyes widen as though I've just invited Paige on a narrowboat holiday.

As Paige talks, I scribble down the worst story I've ever heard in my fifteen-minute-long psychiatric career: one of horrific neglect and every category of abuse by her father. 'But things got really, *really* bad when—'

'OK, thank you Paige,' says Dr Glick as though curbing a child who's eaten too many Skittles. 'Are you on any medications? Do you have any allergies?'

Paige's eyes are glazed from the talk of her early life and what would have turned into full-blown tears retreat to the mysterious reservoir where liquid pain, joy and sentiment reside. Dr Glick returns her stare as empathically as a gargoyle.

'Er, no allergies. Just me methadone, antidepressants, anti-psychotic at night, and my diazepam which keeps me numb.'

Ah, a detective's clue, an open window, a loose hair. 'Paige, why would you want to stay *numb*?' I ask.

'It stops the pain. And without meds I get the flashbacks,' her voice breaking.

'Don't cry Paige,' interjects Dr Glick. 'Do you have any medical problems, high blood pressure, diabetes?'

Dr Glick runs through her list of questions like someone doing a supermarket shop. Fruit and veg aisle first, then bakery, then dairy, and so on. She gives the strong sense that patients are like unruly toddlers who run around picking up things she doesn't want.

'Well I've bashed me head a few times, few bleeds on the brain. Just broken bones really. I think I broke a rib last night. These painkillers are doing nothing, can I get something stronger?'

'What drugs do you use?' asks Dr Glick.

'I never said I use drugs.'

Paige sighs in the silence left for her and looks down at her browned, nicotine-stained fingers. 'Well I suppose heroin, a bit of crack, charlie sometimes, weed if someone's got it. But I'd *never* use meth,' she says with the authority of someone who knows the line.

'I see,' says Glick.

Paige laughs to reveal darkened teeth. 'On the streets smack-heads always joked about how la di da, posh doctors with happy families say "I see", "I know", "I understand". But how d'you? No offence,' she adds.

'If we can return to the psychiatric interview please,' says Dr Glick, 'have you ever been to prison?'

'I don't wanna talk about it.'

'I read you were convicted for GBH assaulting your father.'

'Wouldn't you if you saw him walking down the street like

nothing had happened? Now are you gunna get me something for my ribs?'

'Are you registered with a London GP?' continues Dr Glick. It's as though she's got her frozen items and is heading straight for the checkout.

'Seriously fuck this!' Paige shouts. 'I'm done. Can you even hear me? You lot never help. My ribs fuckin' kill.'

'If you insist on using abusive language I'll have to terminate this interview,' says Dr Glick with infuriating calmness.

'Don't worry, I'm just going to kill myself.'

'Are you really though Paige?' volleys back Dr Glick. 'Because I know from your notes that you say this a lot in A&Es and you're still here,' she adds, like a dissatisfied schoolteacher. Must try harder.

Paige swings her legs to the side and hops off the bed.

'Go if you insist,' says Dr Glick, standing aside. 'Just one more thing so we've covered all bases,' she says, channelling her inner Columbo. 'You told the nurses you were thinking of jumping out of your bedroom window, what floor flat do you live on?'

'Second,' says Paige picking up her plastic bags of belongings.

'Oh fine,' says Dr Glick. 'Goodbye.'

I obediently follow Dr Glick's thin frame back to her office feeling utterly confused. Despite my early feelings about Dom, from reading his assessment earlier he seemed to have the makings of a fairly caring psychiatrist. And if I'd been on-call last night I definitely wouldn't have done anything differently.

Inside Dr Glick's office there are no plants, photos or pictures. The room is as empty as the suicide-proof bedrooms of the patients but for her chunky computer monitor which she gestures for me to document our assessment on.

'There's no true mental illness there,' Dr Glick says, peering over me at the blinking cursor on my empty page. 'It's all just personality disorder and drug-seeking behaviour and there are no wonder drugs for that.'

'Um, could her impulsivity not be a feature of ADHD?' I say, still scrambling to make a good impression.

'She's not posh enough. Maybe if she'd been born on a different *kind* of estate her mummy and daddy could buy her a lovely shiny ADHD diagnosis from Harley Street. But this is the NHS, and they're not paying us any more, so we just say it how it is. Paige is pure personality disorder.'

The truth bombs are falling fast. So much for the mantra that mental illnesses don't discriminate and affect everyone universally, just as broken legs do. Now I'm learning that social class, and later gender and even race, influence what diagnosis a person is given. As does whether you're assessed by a state or private psychiatrist.

Dr Glick starts pacing around the room, arms behind her back. 'In the notes make sure you put that she used abusive language and self-discharged against medical advice. There's nothing we could do anyway. Won't engage with therapy. Hospital admission will only make her more dependent and institutionalised. She always threatens to jump but never does. And what's the worst that could happen anyway . . . what?'

I realise I've been frowning as I type. I clearly need to work on my poker face.

'Which *floor* she lives on?'

She lets out a deep sigh. 'Ben there'll likely be more than one patient threatening to jump out of their window today. Second floor just doesn't cut it.' I open my notebook grateful for this impromptu teaching session, my pen poised over a new page.

'Ben your main job as a psychiatrist, just as a medical doctor, is to keep your patients alive.'

'Keep patients alive,' I scribble down. Then I underline it.

'If you're on-call and a patient tells you they're suicidal, what should you do?'

I know this one, and I'm pretty sure it will come up in my exams. 'Admit them to hospital for treatment and to keep them safe,' I say.

Dr Glick furrows her brow. 'Admit *all* of them? Where are you going to magic thousands of free hospital beds from?'

On her computer I can see she has 60,000 unread emails with more pinging through every minute, many of them titled 'URGENT'. Her eyes flick from her inbox to me and back again, like someone trying to cross a busy motorway.

'You can only admit the *most* suicidal ones,' she continues. 'It's not uncommon for people to get fleeting suicidal thoughts but that doesn't necessarily mean they will kill themselves or even want to.'

Part of me is relieved. I can relate to those annoying intrusive thoughts, my own voice in my head, when I'm standing on the top of a cliff or as a high-speed train is approaching the platform which says *Do it . . . do it now!* I never want to and I'm relieved to hear that it's not pathological and can just about pass as normal.

'If they're not going to kill themselves imminently, you can discharge them home with the crisis team,' Dr Glick continues.

'But how do you know the difference?' I ask.

'Risk assessment. The bread and butter of psychiatry. Your observations of what they say and how they say it. Their history of mental illness or genuine suicide attempts. If there's any secondary gain for them being in hospital. If there are any protective factors or things that might keep them alive.'

'So there is a science to it?'

'Sort of,' she says. 'Gut instinct too. But it's always the ones you least expect. And patients inevitably slip through the net of even the very best psychiatrists.'

Well that's reassuring. I instantly feel overwhelmingly hot. 'Can we open a window please?'

Dr Glick peers out to the car park six floors below us. 'They don't open up here, to stop people jumping out of them.'

'What, even in the psychiatrists' offices?'

'Especially in the psychiatrists' offices,' she says.

I decide to move us on. 'Did I do OK today?'

'I've seen worse. But we're not here to make friends. Maintain your boundaries. A good psychiatrist isn't liked by their patients. If you are, it means you're not prepared to make the tough decisions.'

I don't write that down, it seems illogical.

'Also, you ask too many irrelevant questions. Get a handle on that.'

'Sorry, I'll try and be faster. Perhaps I could observe you in clinic sometime?' On top of running the ward, Dr Glick is also somehow expected to spend a day a week seeing community patients in clinic.

'If you get on top of your ward jobs, yes.'

Her desk phone rings and when she doesn't answer it her mobile phone starts buzzing which she ignores too. 'Now, the most important thing.' She taps the desk for emphasis. 'You must always put the patient's clustering on Carenotes. If you don't enter a diagnosis, the trust won't get paid.'

'But what if I don't know the diagnosis?' I say.

'Well you just need to put something.'

Despite psychiatry having names for its different conditions and the textbooks leading me to believe that mental health classification is no different from diagnosing asthma or diabetes, I'm already noticing that human suffering seems to come in all shapes and sizes. Paige could potentially have fitted into multiple diagnostic boxes; instead she didn't really fit into any.

'It can always be changed later,' she reassures me.*

Dr Glick's desk phone starts ringing again.

'Alright!' Dr Glick says, slapping her hands on her thighs to signify my supervision is over. 'I'd better take this. Go and ask Blessing who's next to be seen.'

I find Blessing politely explaining to a man with a huge terrifying-looking dog that he's not allowed to bring his huge terrifying-looking dog on to the ward. Given my canine phobia I hang back until he leaves and then join her at the open hatch of the clinical room where she starts administering medications. She hands the next patient in line a paper cup of pills: pinks, whites and blues. He knocks them back with a glass of water then opens his mouth and lifts up his tongue. He's ushered on only when Blessing is content that he's swallowed. Most people are on four times a day, some on five.

The line shuffles forward and Blessing acknowledges me, saying she'll be along soon. As I walk back to the office I see Paige, tears now dried, waiting to be let out of the locked ward.

'Take care of yourself,' I say.

'You're new aren't you?' Paige says. My head must drop because she adds, 'That's not a criticism, by the way.'

Something is bothering me. 'Paige can I ask you something?'

'Yeah.'

'I'm sorry that stuff happened when you were younger. But

---

* It can actually be quite hard to lose some labels. In 2017 an American man with no mental health diagnosis was mistaken for someone else who had schizophrenia. When he told doctors he wasn't who they thought he was, this was taken as evidence of his illness. He was forcibly admitted, medicated and incarcerated for two years before he was eventually believed and released (*Guardian*, 4 August 2021).

your tattoos, I noticed you've got one on your arm that says "Dad"?'

She peers at her bare left arm, stretching the skin to bring it into view. A green-blue 'Dad' in a washed-out heart, to balance the 'Mam' one on the right.

She pauses as she tries to square this circle. 'My dad did those bad things,' she eventually says. 'But he was good in other ways. He's the only one who sent me birthday cards in care. And he's my dad so I'll always sort of love him. Families are complicated, you know?'

'I know,' I say.

I return to the one-bedroom flat that my youngest brother Sam and I have just moved into. My NHS income is more steady than his as a hand-to-mouth self-taught silversmith, which means I pay most of the rent. So I have the bedroom and he sleeps on the single mattress we've squeezed into the cupboard under the stairs like Harry Potter. Being brought up essentially on a building site means that he's unfazed sleeping with his head just below a fuse box.

Me and my brothers have always been physically and emotionally close. Josh, who is four years younger than me, is an artist and lives with his partner ten minutes away. One year below him is Gabe, an eighty-hours-a-week chef, who technically lives just round the corner but actually lives in a restaurant kitchen.

After a long day at work it's nice to return to the sanctuary of home. The only slight problem, and something that the estate agent failed to mention, is that our flat shares a paper-thin wall with Europe's largest bodybuilding gym. And we've already discovered that the beefcakes in there don't put the weights down carefully, even if you ask them nicely.

I enter our yellow-painted kitchen-cum-living-room where Sam is making a start at unpacking the cardboard boxes of our stuff as the banging and crashing from next door reverberates around us.

'Hi Benj. You only getting back now?' he says. 'Mum just messaged me to check you're still alive.'

'I literally spoke to her yesterday.'

'Well, she says you haven't replied to her texts today. She was asking if you'd met anyone nice at work,' he says in a studiously neutral way. My inability to hold down a long-term relationship is a topic of enduring fascination to my family.

'Tell her it didn't feel quite right to ask the patients out on my *first* day.'

He grins. 'And she was saying what's missing in her life is a grandchild . . . ah, the kettle!' He heads over to the sink to fill it. 'Save lots of lives today then?' He corrects himself. 'Sorry, save lots of *minds*?'

'Hundreds,' I joke.

As we drink tea sitting on the floor, I consider telling him that the art of psychiatry seems to be less about saving minds and more about saving bed space and finding good reasons to justify withholding care from the limited pot of NHS resources. 'How can I *not* help you?' being the subtext.

Later that night I can't sleep, but not because of the noise. I've wanted to be a psychiatrist for as long as I can remember, partly motivated by a desire to help people just like Paige to live happier and more fulfilling lives. I had never imagined I'd query the legitimacy of people's suffering, use phrases like 'bed blocker', and only offer them help if jumping from a certain floored window would create a big enough splat.

3

BARBARA

I'm in A&E working my first weekend on-call. I'll come to be here so much that I become part of the lead-weighted furniture.*

I've now picked up from Dr Glick that the job of psychiatry is to return people to what are considered 'normal' parameters of human thought, behaviour or emotion. So, for depressed patients, trying to elevate their mood. And for others to try and move it the other way although this model could seem counter-intuitive I thought when my first referral came in.

'I need an urgent psych review for a manic patient who I'm really worried about,' the student nurse in A&E had said. 'She says she's ten out of ten on a happiness scale, walking on cloud nine, says she's never felt better.'

'Oh that doesn't sound right at all,' I'd heard myself replying. 'Yes I'll come and see if we can get her back to normal.'†

Before hanging up I seek to clarify some details. 'Is she on drugs? . . . OK, probably not that then. Is there a known history of mania? . . . Nope, OK. Oh, you say she's *American*. Yes that

---

* Furniture in A&E, just as on psychiatric wards, is lead-weighted to stop patients occasionally throwing it at our heads.

† Bipolar, previously called manic depression, is a label that some people seem happy to use informally about themselves or even keen to formally acquire, due to its association with troubled geniuses like Robin Williams, Stephen Fry or Vincent Van Gogh. But links between madness and creativity are romanticised and you certainly don't need to chop your ear off to be a good artist. Often a true bipolar illness is *unhelpful*, and I never noticed art-talent scouts flocking to Daffodil Ward's art therapy group.

could be it I suppose . . . oh but you say she's flown over here to marry Harry Styles? See you shortly.'

'Barbara Avery?' I say now into the crowded waiting room in a voice which is hopefully starting to sound less unsure of itself.

A woman jumps up from her chair and bounds over to greet me. 'Good morning Doctor. It's so nice to see you!'

I briefly wonder if we've met somewhere before and I out-stretch my hand to buy time. Not content with this formality, and before I have time to react, she plants a big fat kiss on my cheek.

'These are for you,' she says, thrusting a bouquet of hospital-issue flowers into my hand, and I follow her down the corridor to A&E's psychiatric room with her telling me, 'Your eyes look so blue today Doctor, they really pop!'

I realise I've never met Barbara before in my life.

She makes herself comfortable in my swivel chair and starts reading her notes on the computer screen. 'Barbara Avery, 12 March 1966 . . .'

'Um Barbara why don't we swap places? That's usually where the psychiatrist sits.'

'Don't worry I already know everything about psychiatry as some people think I have two brains. Now sit down,' she says, gesturing to the empty chair beside her, 'and I'll teach *you* about psychiatry.'

Her speech is rich and rapid, the words falling from her mouth like coins from a fruit machine. Caught up in her whirl of energy I give up, lay the flowers on the desk and go and sit in the patient's seat. I try to reestablish some power but it's hard when *I'm* now trapped in the corner, furthest away from the door. I rattle off my little spiel about the student-nurses' concerns.

The police had brought Barbara in under a Section 136, a piece of mental health law that enables them to take someone from a public place for an urgent psychiatric review, after she approached them in a London train station at 7 a.m. dressed for her big day asking for directions to St Paul's Cathedral. The ceremony with the One Direction heart-throb wasn't until 3 p.m. and they assured her that if nothing was felt to be wrong, she'd be free to leave in time to say 'I do'.

She had somehow got through a transatlantic flight and customs without anyone seeing anything untoward about a middle-aged woman in a bridal gown telling fellow passengers she was flying to London to marry *Glamour* magazine's sixth-sexiest man in the world. Maybe they just put it down to American self-confidence. Sitting together now, I imagine her trying desperately not to spill the inflight meal down herself.

'Hmm . . . right . . . interesting . . . very interesting,' Barbara says earnestly as I list the police's concerns. She's clicking the end of my retractable pen in and out, a cartoonish impression of a psychiatrist which is actually pretty good.

'Right,' she says ignoring everything I've said. 'The first thing you need to know about psychiatry, is that it doesn't actually exist. There's no actual evidence for any of it. It's just social control. I've read Thomas Szasz and *The Myth of Mental Illness*. You modern shrinks might have abolished the asylums and stopped drilling holes into people's heads and mushing up their brains with ice picks. But now your patients are just zombies in chemical straightjackets aren't they?'

I've been learning about these famous anti-psychiatrists such as Thomas Szasz, R. D. Laing and Erving Goffman for the 'history of psychiatry' component of my exams. They query the scientific rigour of psychiatry's so-called 'illnesses' and the profession's licence to do things to people which outside a psychiatric hospital would constitute human rights abuses.*

It's weird partly agreeing with someone dressed in a meringue wedding dress who claims to be marrying Harry Styles. But if I admit that to Barbara I'll lose whatever scrap of credibility I still have with her.

'Barbara thank you for the flowers,' I say trying to move us on, 'but honestly you shouldn't have.' I've noticed that doctors get given fewer gifts working in psychiatry, and when you do get one, you worry. 'Have you been buying lots of presents lately?' I ask, a common feature of mania being overspending.†

'What does it matter if I have? Money is just paper isn't it? That's why I flew business class. And everyone's planting more trees these days so we'll never run out!'

The problem is that sometimes during manic episodes, patients can do things which they later regret. Dr Glick has told me about patients going on reckless credit-card-funded spending sprees and buying three Lamborghinis, £10,000-worth of ice sculptures which have melted into the carpet by the morning, or withdrawing all their money and throwing it off the top of the Tate gallery to make it rain cash.

I write 'overspending' in my notebook and move us on to

---

* Psychiatry is the only medical speciality with a flourishing 'Survivor Movement' stemming not from its ailments (like cancer survivors) but its very treatments and practices. It is also unique in having an entire movement devoted to its abolition, in the form of the Anti-Psychiatry Movement. For example, there's no Anti-Dermatology Movement and it's hard to imagine people ever protesting in the streets against the evils of E45 emollient cream.

† If you're reading this book with forty-nine other copies sitting next to you following a manic spending spree, please go to A&E immediately. But maybe leave an online review on Amazon or Goodreads first.

another potentially worrying symptom. 'Barbara, would you tell me about your relationship with Harry Styles?'

'You can just call him Harry,' she says. 'Well it was love at first sight for both of us. You know when you just know?'

I don't know. I'm not really the person to consult on love. But this sounds very much like the sort of thing my parents and grandparents always say about the first time they met.

Barbara looks longingly at her screensaver; a photo of a topless Harry Styles lying in white bedsheets, looking down a camera lens. It's the sort of shot that could only be taken by a lover, or a *GQ* magazine photographer.

She tells me that Harry Styles first declared his love for her in Connecticut during One Direction's world tour. He had gazed out to the capacity crowd but there was only one person he looked at like that. The decisive factor for Barbara was that at the exact same moment Harry had looked at her, he'd run his fingers through his hair. That was the code.

I suspect Barbara is manic with erotomania, a delusional disorder whereby people develop the unshakable belief that someone of high status is, pardon the phrase, madly in love with them.*

She says since that first encounter Harry Styles has been communicating via tweets, song lyrics and YouTube videos. He proposed when during a music video he wore a yellow jumper which is her favourite colour and spoke about birthdays which

---

* In an early case of erotomania a woman stood for hours outside Buckingham Palace believing any twitching of the curtains was King George V communicating his secret love for her. The objects of such patients' affections are typically rich, famous, powerful or high-status: actors, musicians, professors, politicians and sometimes even doctors. Presumably not NHS doctors, though.

meant they should wed on her sixtieth. Sure enough her date of birth on the A&E notes corresponds with today's date. 'Happy birthday,' I say struggling to sound excited for her.

Barbara doesn't consider it odd that she's never actually met her supposed husband-to-be, that they live thousands of miles apart or that according to tabloids, Harry Styles is in a romantic relationship with Taylor Swift.

'Some people might think,' I begin tactfully ('some people' is a helpful phrase I've picked up from Dr Glick, which is a less confrontational way of saying 'I'), 'that Harry Styles touching his hair or wearing yellow don't necessarily mean that he loves and wants to marry you. What would you say to them?'

'I'd say they know jack shit. It's a feeling.' She tilts her head to the side sympathetically. 'You've never been in love before have you?'

I flinch.

'This isn't really about me,' I say, a neat deflection that psychiatrists can use which unfortunately doesn't work in quite the same way with my own mum. I decide to move us on. 'Isn't Harry Styles going out with a famous pop star?'

Her tone changes. 'Taylor? It's a sham relationship for the papers. He despises her!'

She volunteers that she's booked a hotel for tonight for them to consummate the marriage, and asks if I've heard of it, a place called the Travelodge.

I'm learning that psychiatrists need to keep an open mind. Stranger things have happened than celebrities meeting mystery older women in budget hotels. And not everything psychiatric patients say is unreliable.

Recently on Daffodil Ward a hospitalised man asked for leave so he could visit the Queen. Dr Glick had swiftly rejected his request, interpreting it as a grandiose delusion to go with all his other ones. It later transpired that the patient had actually been awarded an MBE and left Her Majesty waiting.

'OK, let's try and imagine every possibility. What if Harry doesn't come to the cathedral?'

'I'd go to his house because I'd know that trailer-trash Taylor was preventing him from meeting me.'

Uh-oh.

'And would you just be wanting to have a chat or—'

'I'd fucking kill her!' Just in case something is lost in translation, she slides a finger across her neck.

Oh God.

Whether or not Barbara means this figuratively, I think I might be saved by a practical hurdle in her way. 'But I don't suppose you actually know where Harry Styles lives?'

'Of course I do,' she snaps. 'He left it on the Internet for me. It's where I send all his gifts and letters. The ones that that hoe intercepts.' Barbara unlocks her mobile and enters an address from memory into Google maps; 'It's close, 1.7 miles away, so just a thirty-five-minute walk.'

Maybe more if you're wearing heels, I think.

I imagine Barbara turning up at Harry Styles's luxury home. Delusions are by definition unshakable, so all signs would only ever point to his undying love for her. Even if standing on his doorstep while holding hands with his A-list partner he shouted, 'I don't love you Barbara, now get the fuck off my property!' she'd likely respond, 'Oh Harry, that's such a you thing to say.'

Barbara won't come into hospital voluntarily but she's made some alarming comments which could endanger Taylor Swift or even Harry Styles. There's two people I never thought I'd have to worry about today.

The Mental Health Act is the legal framework that allows people who are considered a danger to themselves or others to be brought into hospital and even given treatment against their will. 'Sectioning' as its colloquially known is a strange super-power that requires two senior independent psychiatrists and a nurse or social worker all to agree. This is to safeguard abuses of the past where a single psychiatrist could indefinitely commit someone to an asylum for the most tenuous of reasons. As a junior, thankfully restricting someone's liberty isn't a responsi-bility that rests on my shoulders, yet.

'Barbara, I'd like you to speak to some of my senior colleagues.' She tries to follow me out of the interview room, but two burly security guards in stab vests stand in her way. She sighs, sits back down and starts playing 'What Makes You Beautiful' through her phone.

I call the on-call senior registrar who agrees to come with the necessary ensemble. I complete my notes then try to read about my next patients amongst the tinny music, beeping machines and phone calls in A&E. From his cubicle, a bedridden elderly man calls out in a thin voice. 'Hello!' he says again when no one comes to his aid. 'Hello?'

All the nurses and health care assistants are occupied. The doc-tors keep their heads lowered, their gazes on their paperwork.

'Help!' the frail man continues. He's fruitlessly pressing his 'assistance' button. 'Please somebody help!'

I go over to assist him and thankfully it's an easy one, he just wants a glass of water. Once I've fetched it, despite his Parkinson-ian tremor he manages to get most of it past his lips.

Later on, when Barbara tries to abscond, security close the door and monitor her through the glass porthole. I'm sitting with a young man who's slit his wrists following a relationship break-up, a more bread-and-butter love-fuelled mental health crisis, when I hear her start to bang on the door.

Eventually, my co-workers arrive, review Barbara, and then

make the necessary arrangements to bring her into hospital. Cruelly, her transport arrives at bang on three o'clock. It's not a horse-drawn carriage or a limousine, but an ambulance to take her to a psychiatric hospital. She's not going quietly and I can hear her screaming 'How can you do this to me, on my wedding day?!' I apologise to the young man and peer out from our bay's paper curtains at the commotion. After a scuffle, the security guards escort Barbara down the corridor and a procession of nurses follow behind with her belongings, like bridesmaids.

Even though it's not technically me sectioning Barbara I can't help feeling responsible for starting off the chain of events that will not only deprive her of her liberty but also decide what powerful medicines will flow through her veins. There's a long and troubled history too of male doctors incarcerating women in asylums for as little as having a child out of wedlock, masturbating or due to 'hysteria'.[1]

Although I'm pretty sure that Barbara has erotomania, I'm also starting to wonder whether mental illnesses are really as categorical as we make out. It's comforting, and simpler, to pretend that someone either has depression or schizophrenia or bipolar or erotomania, or they don't. 8 billion people boiled down into two camps of sane or insane.

I sense in reality these concepts are more dimensional and on a spectrum. For example, how accurate can any of us be about another person's true feelings towards us?

Over our snatched canteen lunches Nafisa constantly tries to decipher cryptic texts from her boyfriend, seemingly unsure of his true feelings, despite him saying he wants to spend the rest of his life with her.

On the train down to the capital to start working as a psychiatrist I thought I had a strong connection with the attractive woman I was sitting next to. As we spoke and laughed I imagined our future lives together (would I move back to Newcastle or would she come down to London?) right until the point she mentioned her fiancé and forthcoming maternity leave.

Growing up, I saw people harm each other in ways that some might argue de facto excludes the presence of love. If my own parents are delusional about the presence of love that isn't really there, do they have erotomania too?

These are the thoughts whizzing through my mind after work in the supermarket. As I peruse the aisles, I notice the domestic scenes around me. A mother pushing a trolley around with a toddler who's being placated with some Pom Bears. A young, contented couple are silently adding ingredients to a shared basket for a recipe that they'll cook together later.

I've got a tension headache, perhaps from the stress, ward noise and bright computer screens, so into my basket I also stock up on painkillers.

'I'm not allowed to sell you three packets of paracetamols,'* says the no-nonsense cashier in her company-issue fleece.

I'm tired and I've got a splitting headache. 'Why not?' I ask grumpily.

'Supermarket policy. Also, for all I know you could be going to kill yourself tonight.'

I've never been suicidal before and I look at my other items on the conveyor belt. A kilogram box of Sugar Puffs. Some UHT milk. And one of those large jars of Marmite that takes about ten

---

* Restrictions on pack sizes and over-the-counter sales have actually significantly reduced fatalities from paracetamol overdoses. Having to visit multiple shops to stockpile the necessary quantities buys time for impulsive suicidal feelings to pass and a person to have second thoughts.

years to get through. Maybe still eating Sugar Puffs at my age could be seen as a red flag, but does she really think this is my strange last meal?

I want to say to her 'I'm clearly not going to do anything *tonight*. For one thing it's long-life milk.'

I reluctantly hand over one of the packets and just to see the look on her face I consider asking if I could swap them for some bleach or razor blades.

Back at home, the flat is cold and empty, Sam still in his workshop. Not even the crashing of dumbbells or grunting men next door for company. I unpack my shopping from the carrier bag and check my phone. No texts, not even from my mum.

Nobody likes you. Why don't you put that plastic bag over your head?

Thanks for that, brain. It unhelpfully throws me this stuff sometimes, but at least I now know from Dr Glick that I'm *fine*. I sit down at the kitchen table with my tea, toast and Marmite. As I eat, I read the back of the food packets, a comforting habit I've had since childhood, where my mind can escape into nutritional information.

Next to the Utterly Butterly customer services phone number, in a friendly font is written 'Fancy a chat?', and a small part of me genuinely considers calling.

4

GLADYS

'Should we catch up?' Dr Glick says on Monday morning.

We're supposed to meet for a protected hour once a week to take stock and reflect on what we're doing here. But because there's never enough time, so far we've only managed one at the end of my first week, for thirteen minutes. I nod, try to swallow a yawn and follow her sleepily into her office.

'So how are things?' she says closing the door. Things.

Should I tell her about how uncomfortable I felt triggering Barbara's section and depriving her of her liberty? Or of how disturbingly quickly I seem to have slipped into casually dismissing 'the regulars' who clog up my out-of-hours shifts? Or ask why, since there's no ward psychologist for talking therapy, we don't just fill a vending machine with antidepressants and antipsychotics? When I recently complained to Blessing about this she'd patted my arm and said, 'Benjamin it must be really difficult for *you*.'

But instead I just tell her I'm a bit tired trying to find my feet on Daffodil Ward. Taking all the bloods, ordering and chasing investigations, assessing new admissions, taking more bloods. Plus all the on-calls on top of trying to revise for exams.

Dr Glick nods to convey empathy. I imagine she learnt that at a training day. 'Why did you choose to specialise in psychiatry, Ben?' she asks.

Do not, whatever you do, mention your parents.

This is somewhat out of the blue and the first time she's ever shown any curiosity in me. 'I dunno really, I've just always felt drawn to it,' I say.

She leans back in her chair, hugging a mug on her desk with both hands to signify that she's got all day. And I know better than to play silence-chicken with a psychiatrist. After a noble resistance of seven or eight seconds I tell her 'Maybe it's because psychiatrists get to retire five years earlier than the other medical specialities.'

She narrows her eyes. 'You do know that's only because we're statistically more likely to burn out and kill ourselves, right?'*

No, I definitely didn't know that.

'Plus they scrapped that scheme years ago,' she adds. Dr Glick takes a sip from her mug and winces at what is clearly cold coffee. 'Are you in therapy?' she asks.

'No!' I say, as though she's just asked me to describe my favourite sexual position.

'Well, I'm supposed to tell you that you should be. People are still bashful about it over here but in America every man and his dog is in therapy. Quite literally, CBT for dogs is a thing now.'

I consider making a joke about how does that work when they're not allowed on the couch, but manage to stop myself.

'I usually recommend it to trainees. Especially if they're committing their life to something and don't know why,' she gives me what I realise is a smile. It's a bit like she's had it explained to her in an instruction manual, but at least she's trying. 'I could recommend my old therapist if you like?'

'*You've* had therapy?' I say, failing to hide my surprise. Dr Glick seems indestructible.

'Of course. The GMC's code of practice requires us to look after ourselves so we can care for our patients. It also helps when

---

* Psychiatrists, I now know, have notoriously high levels of mental illness, substance misuse problems and suicide. On the life expectancy tables I think they're just above shark tamer but just below Vladimir Putin's food taster.

patients say *you're* mad and that you need help, because you can tell them that you're getting it.'

'But, I'm *fine*,' I protest, probably too much. I just can't always sleep, grind my teeth and sometimes wake up screaming like everyone else.

'Maybe,' says Dr Glick. 'But there is something odd about picking this speciality; why would anyone in their right mind *choose* to spend their working life around human distress? There's no shame in mental health professionals needing mental health professionals, just as hairdressers need hairdressers. If we all cut our own hair, it would be a mess!'

My family are exactly the type of people who cut their own hair. Damn she's good.

'Psychiatrists used to get therapy for free but you know, cuts. Tell him I sent you and he may offer low-fee sessions.' She writes something on a scrap of paper and hands it to me. 'Now, shall we crack on and see the new admissions?' I look at the clock. Thirteen minutes.

Sitting upright on the edge of her hospital bed, Gladys stares ahead as though expecting a bus. Despite the room being a usual hospital swelter, she won't take her duffel coat off because she's cold. Oh, and she claims to be dead.

'Gladys you don't look very comfortable,' I say, standing beside Dr Glick. 'Your daughter says you've not slept for a week. Maybe lie down and get some rest.'

'I'll lie down when you take me to the graveyard,' she mutters.

She's perhaps not far off meeting her maker. Her well-worn coat appears too big, as under it she is worryingly thin. Her sallow skin is only one shade pinker than my medical-school cadaver 'Clive', and pulled tight across her skull like cellophane.

No one looks their best in a psychiatric hospital and I squint to try and see the person beneath her illness. I can just about imagine her as the kind-hearted science teacher she reportedly was, telling children not to run in the corridors.

Gladys recently alarmed her daughter by voicing that her organs were in the wrong places. Her heart was where her lungs should be, her brain was jammed in her womb, and her guts were in her head. Unsurprisingly, she was brought to A&E.

Because she wasn't drinking, her electrolytes were deranged (it's still OK to call extreme levels of sodium and potassium that, just not people), but other examinations and investigations were normal. It was official: Gladys wasn't 100%, she was malnourished and dehydrated, but her organs were in the right places and she was certainly alive.* So she was sectioned and transferred to 'the other hospital', hidden behind the main one.

Dr Glick notes the untouched water jug on the bedside table. 'Gladys you need to drink some fluids.'

'Dead people don't drink,' Gladys says staring straight ahead at the wall.

Dr Glick coughs. 'I don't think your antidepressants are

---

* Medical students spend five years learning to discern the living from the dead, but sometimes even that isn't enough. A Polish woman started moving in the morgue after eleven hours in cold storage, then went home for some soup to warm up. (BBC, 2014.) Perhaps the closest shave came for a Venezuelan man who woke up on the cold slab of a pathologist's table just as he was being acquainted with an autopsy knife. His grieving wife turned up to identify the body and was dumbfounded to find him waiting for her in the corridor. (Reuters, 2017.)

working. So we're going to have to try something else. Starting from this afternoon.'

Striding out and back down the long, corridor Dr Glick says to me, 'She was saying that in A&E. It's classic Cotard's syndrome, you're lucky to see it.'* We enter the nursing office and sit down. 'She needs electroconvulsive therapy,' Dr Glick adds.

I nearly laugh but remember that Dr Glick doesn't make jokes.

'Um, do we still do that?' I ask. I know a member of my family had shock therapy, but a long time ago.

She sighs. 'Ben, watch fewer films and read more textbooks. Shock therapy is still one of psychiatry's most effective treatments and works a damn sight faster than drugs. She'll die if she doesn't start drinking. Unless you have any better ideas? Any miracle new psychiatric cures you're not telling me about?'

I look down at the floor.

'Luckily Dr Cerletti has agreed to squeeze her onto his ECT list today as an emergency.' She sees the look on my face. 'You should go and see it. In fact no, you should *do* it. You need to for your training anyway. So I can sign you off as competent at the end of the year. Do some bloods first. Sunflower Suite, top floor, 5 p.m.'

Sectioning people on Sunday. Shock therapy on Monday. I'll be waterboarding someone by Tuesday.

I grudgingly collect blood bottles, needles and a tourniquet

---

* Cotard's, or Walking Corpse syndrome, is a rare delusional disorder where the patient believes they're dead, have lost their internal organs or are rotting. In one early case, the sufferer demanded she be dressed and laid to rest. Without any better ideas in 1788 her family dutifully complied and even put on a sham funeral, not that it appeased her. Lying in her open coffin she complained that her shroud was the wrong colour.

from the clinical room, then optimistically look in the dining room for Gladys. Spring sunshine bathes the patients as they eat with plastic cutlery at their bolted-down tables. Staff members hover in the doorway, observing, so the patients eat silently and self-consciously, yet as 'normally' as possible, aware that any false move – trying to eat soup with a fork, buttering both sides of their toast or forgetting to peel a banana before eating it – may be reported back to Dr Glick and risk extending their stay. The only noise is from the ladies serving lunch and a new manic patient who hasn't yet got the memo who's singing 'Jingle Bells' between mouthfuls. It's April. No sign of Gladys though.

I go to her room via the kitchen. If I can get her to eat and drink we can call the whole thing off. As the kettle boils I wonder how it could be therapeutic to jolt with electricity that 1.5 kg jelly blob between our ears.

'Mind if I come in?' I say, a cup of tea in each hand. I put them down and reveal a plastic-wrapped sandwich from each of my back pockets. 'I thought I'd do room service!'

Gladys is in exactly the same position she was twenty minutes ago. Textbook catatonia.

'I should introduce myself properly, I'm Benjamin one of the doctors,' I say, pulling up a chair. 'There's ham or cheese and tomato. Which one do you fancy Gladys? Gladys?'

I try a different tack and take a big gulp of tea, swallowing with a satisfied 'Ahhhhhh,' as though trying to coax a toddler to finish their Fruit Shoot.

Next I try silence, which most people find so intolerable they feel compelled to fill, like when people whistle in lifts. Maybe I'm putting too much pressure on her though. I relax back into my chair, look out of the window and consider the afternoon ahead.

Dare I conscientiously object, or just like participants in that infamous study* will I obey the lab coat authority figure and deliver electric shocks to the brain; the most sensitive computer system in the universe?

After ten minutes, and already behind with my ward jobs, I give up. 'Right Gladys, I'll get out of your hair,' I say picking up her cold tea. 'Keep the sandwiches, just in case.' And then a result, of sorts.

'Dead people don't eat,' she whispers.

I sit back down again and try appealing to her rational mind. 'Gladys, your daughter said you used to be a biology teacher?'

'Until I retired.'

'My dad was briefly too!' I say, clawing for some connection but nothing registers on her face. It's not the best story, to be fair. 'So you taught biology, the study of living things?' She nods. 'But if you're dead, how do you explain talking to me now?'

She ponders this for a moment. 'You must be dead too.'

What a way to find out. Also, it certainly won't reflect well on me, if in the afterlife I am still working in the NHS.

Accepting defeat, I apply the tourniquet, hit one of her thin, wriggly veins with my needle and thick crimson floods the chamber. As I wait for the bottles to fill, I wonder if I'm in a strange dream. But as I exit Gladys's room the glass bottles I'm now

---

* In the 1960s Stanley Milgram investigated whether 'obedience' could explain how atrocities like the Holocaust could be committed by ordinary people. The study's participants were 'teachers' asking questions to a 'learner' strapped to an electric chair (the 'learner' was actually an actor, and the electrodes weren't really live). When the 'learner' invariably gave an incorrect answer, the participant was instructed by a lab-coat-wearing 'experimenter' to administer increasingly powerful electric shocks from 15 to 450 volts. Despite the actor begging, screaming and later even becoming unresponsive, all participants went up to 300 volts, and two-thirds to what would have been a deadly 450 volts.

clutching are a welcome reality test. I can see her dark red blood in the tubes. And what's more, I can feel its warmth in my palm.

Now *I* can't stomach my canteen meal deal. Whenever I look at the prawns in my sandwich, I see mini-cerebrums. Just before 5 p.m. I head to the Sunflower Suite, which is signposted above its doorframe in a jolly Comic Sans font.

Inside the waiting room of magnolia walls, classical music plays on the radio with Gladys sitting in a hospital bed wearing an NHS gown. A no-nonsense anaesthetist from over the road, dressed in scrubs and surgical clogs, is trying to insert a cannula but Gladys is explaining that she doesn't have any blood vessels in her body, and based on the anaesthetist's troubled expression I sense there's a reason he chose to specialise in putting patients to sleep.

A nurse on the other side of the bed going through a checklist looks up at me. 'Dr Cerletti is getting everything ready in the Recovery Room,' she says.

'Come in! Come in!' says the short, animated fellow zealously fiddling with the buttons of the barbecue-sized ECT machine. I'm half-surprised it bears no cartoonish 'Danger – High Voltage' sticker. To complete the Mad Professor look, he too has wild, unruly hair as though he's had some shock therapy himself.

'You must be Benjamin.'

'Yes, hello Dr Cerletti.'

'Thanks for doing her work-up, bloods weren't too bad!' he says jovially. 'Some acute kidney failure but that's not surprising given the poor thing is as dry as a tax return. Dr Glick said you'd like to do this one?'

I definitely never said that.

Playing the enthusiastic new trainee, I don't disagree.

He's like an excitable Curry's shop assistant as he proudly

shows me the leads, screen and electrodes of the latest model. He's already completed the prescription chart where instead of a drug and a dose in milligrams the 'medicine' is written as a strength and duration of electrical current.

'Any questions before we go through?' says Dr Cerletti.

'This is probably a stupid one, but how does ECT work?'

'Nobody knows,' he says with a wry smile. 'One of life's big mysteries. But it's a bit like switching a frozen computer on and off again.'

Ah, that highly scientific technique.

'Do you know the history of ECT?'

I shake my head.

'Shock treatments' origins stem from early observations by the Greeks and Hippocrates that people's madness *improved* following an epileptic fit. So from the late 1930s physicians sought to induce fits artificially with chemicals and later with electricity. And here we are.'

'Wow, right. And um, why's the anaesthetist here?'

He looks at me puzzled. 'To administer the general anaesthetic of course. You didn't think we'd give ECT *awake*?'

I don't want to admit that until now my sole knowledge of electroconvulsive therapy has come from the film *One Flew Over the Cuckoo's Nest.*

'Originally, patients were conscious for ECT but as anaesthetics developed patients could be put to sleep first.' Shaking his head he adds, 'Dear me this isn't the s . . .' and I think he's about to say Stone Age but he ends with '. . . sixties.'

He pushes the machine through the swing doors, parks it behind Gladys's head, then plugs it into the mains.

The anaesthetist lowers Gladys flat and applies an oxygen mask. Then he injects a muscle relaxant which Dr Cerletti whispers to me is to make her go floppy and prevent any 'unwanted fractures' from the fitting. Then he injects the milky anaesthetic propofol. 'This is the pina colada,' the anaesthetist says, a stock line that doesn't get the polite smile it likely does at the general hospital. 'Imagine you're relaxing on a white sandy beach,' he continues to no reaction at all. 'We'll see you in half an hour!'

With Gladys now out cold we wash our hands at the sink with splodges of pink surgical soap, as Dr Cerletti whistles like a tradesman about to renovate someone's loft.

'Benjamin some medics say they'd never choose psychiatry because you don't save lives. But in this ECT suite I've saved *hundreds*.' Drying his hands with paper towels he adds, 'On the trolley you'll find the bite-block – it'll stop her biting her tongue or shattering her teeth during the seizure – yes that's the one.'

I prise Gladys's dry lips open and fix the rubber structure in place.

'OK we're ready . . . Benjamin apply the electrodes!'

I hesitate; am I really going to do this?

'Preferably before the propofol runs out,' snarks the anaesthetist who is ventilating our patient with a bag and mask.

Everything feels tighter; my elbows seem to be banging against the others around the bedside. We are packed in so tight I can smell the anaesthetist's coffee breath.

'Benjamin?' says Dr Cerletti.

I do as I'm told, trying to steady my hands as I place the paddles on Gladys's temples. The incongruous tinkling of piano keys and romantic strings are still coming from the radio. Then Dr Cerletti presses the red button.

I await the sparks, bolts of electricity zigzagging through the air, violent open-eyed convulsions and jaw-clamping with enough force to snap wooden spoons. But it doesn't happen. Gladys's closed eyelids tighten as if she's just accidentally rinsed shampoo into them. Her jaw digs into the jelly guard. Her body stiffens but there are no convulsions. Within a minute it's over, and her body relaxes back into the bed. The orchestral score on the radio also winds down, there's a moment of silence, and then the honey-voiced Classic FM disc jockey is jabbering away again.

Dr Cerletti prints off a paper electroencephalogram (EEG) trace showing brainwave activity and holds it up triumphantly. 'Oh look at that, it's a beauty! Well done team! An *excellent* seizure!'

Having never celebrated a seizure before, I'm not familiar with the etiquette. Should I clap? The nurse and anaesthetist simply wheel Gladys into the Recovery Room to wake up following her cerebral 'control, alt, delete' treatment.

'Will she be OK?' I ask.

'She should be fine,' says Dr Cerletti. 'She'll come round in about fifteen minutes.' He glances at the clock on the wall; it's nearly six o'clock. 'You get off early Benjamin, I'll do the paperwork. We'll drop her at the ward later.'

Back home, I have the flat to myself. Sam and I have now unboxed everything in the living area and we've sorted out our bedrooms too. Admittedly his didn't take very long.

I'm reading *Madness in Civilization* by the sociologist and researcher Andrew Scull for the 'history of psychiatry' module of my exams. It seems that the experience of human suffering has remained an unavoidable constant throughout time. But how we conceptualise it, what we call it, and how we try to manage it has changed.

Treatments for madness, as mental illness was previously known, have included: drilling a hole in the head so the evil could 'escape'; dropping caged patients into freezing water until they nearly drowned to 'shock' them out of their illness as if curing a case of hiccups; rotating patients incredibly fast on a spinning chair; removing bodily parts such as teeth, tonsils, colons and cervixes thought to be the infective site of madness; injecting patients with cyanide, malaria or huge doses of insulin to induce coma; inserting an ice-pick-like object via the eye socket to mush up the brain. At the time, each of these treatments was heralded as a miracle cure; Egas Moniz, the pioneer of lobotomy, was even awarded a Nobel Prize in Medicine in 1949. But their benefits had been overplayed and their harms minimised and such practices have now been abolished. Only ECT continues, despite much controversy. Although there is some evidence of its efficacy, I've also read that interestingly many patients also improve after having 'sham ECT' (a placebo equivalent where you're put to sleep, then on waking you're told you were given ECT when you weren't), and slightly worryingly the pro-ECT research hasn't been repeated since the 1980s. Critics also cite long-term harms such as headaches, memory loss and, at its worst, lasting brain damage.

'See anything interesting today then Benj?' Sam asks when he gets in.

Putting a human computer on and off again seems embarrassingly crude to explain. Plus I'm still not sure how I feel about today. I'm reminded of another concept I've learnt about while revising for my exams: the Dunning–Kruger effect, the unsettling phenomenon which means that the more I seem to learn, the less I feel I know.

It's unnerving to think that at so many points in history psychiatrists have practised in ways that they believed were helpful for their patients, only for such practices to later be debunked as pseudoscience, or worse, barbarism.

I snap my book shut. This is why people just watch TV.

'Nah, not really,' I say. 'Let's watch *Come Dine with Me*.'

Sam flops onto the sofa with me and tries to turn on the television. When the remote control doesn't work, he bangs it hard on his hand until it does. I wonder if that'll be tomorrow's approach if Gladys hasn't improved.

The next morning, I head straight to Gladys's bedroom. It's empty. Shit.

I burst into the office. 'Where's Gladys?'

Blessing looks up from reading about the overnight admissions. 'Good morning to you too. She's in the dining room.'

'What?'

'Gladys is in the dining room.'

'What's she doing there?'

Blessing looks at me quizzically. 'What do you think?'

I follow the smell of bacon down the corridor to the dining area. There's a queue of patients lining up at the hotplate for porridge or a cooked breakfast. An untouched fruit bowl sits on the side.

And there, alone at a table with that unmistakably straight spine, is Gladys. She still looks emaciated now back in her duffel coat. But in front of her is a nearly-empty beaker of apple juice and, but for a residual baked-bean puddle, a clean plate.

A single case study hardly proves that ECT 'works', and on Daffodil Ward I will see plenty of instances when it does nothing at all. But it worked for Gladys, for now. No one knows why, but it seems you've just got to take what you can get in this mysterious speciality. First, do no harm. Second, somehow do some good. Third, make sure you enter a diagnostic code so the trust gets paid.

5

ANTON

A receptionist pokes her head into Dr Glick's bare office. 'Your two o'clock has just cancelled. Apparently his house is flooding,' she says before disappearing.

'OK Ben,' says Dr Glick unable to hide her delight, 'I'm just going to catch up with some emails.' She turns to her inbox and I remember she's got 60,000 to get through.

Several months into the job on Daffodil Ward, she's letting me observe some of her outpatient clinics. I'm getting faster and each day I see new admissions, take their history, do a mental state examination (MSE) which is like an MOT of the mind, do a physical and take blood to rule out any organic problems. Then I'll choose a diagnosis, enter the appropriate 'cluster' in the system, the wide diversity of human experience reduced to a simple code containing a letter and some numbers, and then Dr Glick initiates treatment.

The patients are like fruit on a processing line, only instead of those little sticky labels that go on apples, oranges and bananas, our bestsellers are schizophrenia, bipolar, depression and emotionally unstable personality disorder.

Dr Glick has taught me that the trick is simply to note the presence or absence of key symptoms – like low or elated mood, auditory or visual hallucinations, persecutory or grandiose delusions – and not to get bogged down in the so-called 'personal history' which is their life story.

I'm now more confident on night shifts when assessing patients alone. I'm getting better at winning favour with my seniors by finding creative ways to not admit patients: wrong postcode, too physically unwell to accept on to a psychiatric ward, a suspected diagnosis of 'just' personality disorder, or the presence of drug and alcohol intoxication which could be mimicking mental illness. I've received only one rude email from an inpatient consultant for 'inappropriately' admitting a homeless man who was saying all the right things and who I couldn't bear to kick out on to the streets at 1 a.m. But perhaps my biggest achievement to date is that recently I said something that Blessing almost found funny.

I've also got a good thing going on with our ward's canteen ladies. Apparently because of health and safety or insurance, staff aren't meant to eat the 6,000 tonnes of untouched hospital food wasted each year. Now, instead of chucking it all away after the patients' lunch, I've persuaded the canteen ladies to carefully stack up the laden takeaway trays in a fresh bin bag for me to feast on when I get a minute. Sometimes when they're exiting the ward they'll wink at me like we're characters in *Ocean's Eleven* performing a heist on a casino vault. Often the highlight of my day is eating a free 'bin lunch' of four vegetable pasties, mash, beans, sponge and chocolate sauce, or whatever is on the menu that day.

This gross food waste, in combination with the impossible-to-turn-off radiators on full blast, doesn't much reassure me about the climate when natural disasters regularly feature on the news: floods, droughts, wildfires. Maybe I needn't worry about the NHS's environmental footprint, though. As commitment to a 'green plan', our trust recently added a leaf to its email footer.

As Dr Glick wades through her emails I take the opportunity to study the *Oxford Handbook of Psychiatry* that I keep in my jacket pocket, its pages becoming well worn, their corners folded.

'What are you reading?' Dr Glick says after a while.

I look up. 'The psychiatric diagnostic systems.'

She raises an eyebrow and keeps typing. 'I think I'll wait for the film.'

Was that a joke from Dr Glick?

Here, like the rest of the UK, we use the ICD-10: the International Classification of Disease, which codes every condition, including mental illnesses. All of them in there together – diabetes, schizophrenia, pulmonary heart disease, all with an alphanumeric code. The codes for the mental and behavioural disorders all begin with the letter F, which may or may not stand for 'fuuuuuuck'.*

It means that after seeing a patient I can never just write 'depression'. I have to decide if it's a mild depressive episode (F32.0), a moderate depressive episode (F32.1), a severe depressive episode without psychotic symptoms (F32.2), a severe depressive episode with psychotic symptoms (F32.3), atypical depression (F32.8), a depressive episode unspecified (F32.9), or recurrent depressive disorder (F33).

At medical school I had wondered why modern medicine continued to adopt highly technical vocabulary when it surely only bamboozled patients until I realised that was partly its function. We're more likely to respect a doctor who diagnoses synchronous diaphragmatic flutters rather than the hiccups.

'Could we quickly go over some treatments?' I ask, trying my luck. Dr Glick clicks her mouse, there's the swooshing sound of an email sending, and she turns back to me. One down, 59,999 to go.

'Go on,' she says.

---

* This is not to be confused with the so called 'bible of psychiatry' the American *Diagnostic and Statistical Manual of Mental Disorders* or *DSM*. Here some psychiatrists first entered conditions into the book based on what they'd seen in their clinical practice. What began in *DSM-1* in 1952 with 106 conditions has now ballooned to more than 400 in *DSM-5*, a Walmart catalogue of every brand of human misery. Slightly alarmingly 69% of those responsible for the latest edition had financial ties to pharmaceutical companies.

'F32.0 . . .'

'Depressive episodes. For clinical depression always start with a selective serotonin reuptake inhibitor. The SSRIs. They're thought to work by correcting chemical imbalances in the brain.'

Makes sense, I think, dutifully noting down the proposed mechanism. 'And when I'm working in the community am I allowed to prescribe them?'

'You're a doctor so prescribing is your job,' she says. 'If you don't then how are you any better than a psychologist?'

I didn't realise that psychologists and psychiatrists were at war with each other. Words versus chemical warfare. My mum versus me.

'Take this,' Dr Glick says, handing me something from her top drawer. 'You'll be needing it when your next job comes around.'

Receiving my own psychiatric prescription pad feels momentous, like the first time you hang a stethoscope around your neck or see 'Dr' on your bank card.

I smile as I run my thumb through the pad's thin pages. Prescriptions are green, the colour of life and growth. And money in cartoons.

As instructed, I go and collect our '2.30' – Anton, a twenty-two-year-old postgraduate art student who was referred by his GP with a list of his problems, which doctors always like to know ahead of time. It's why patients should never google their symptoms, because then it's just duplication of work when doctors do it.

Sitting in the waiting room, his shoulders are hunched forward and his head is covered. I call his name, and he shuffles down the corridor in his scuffed Converse trainers. Inside Dr Glick's consultation room Anton lowers his black hoodie to reveal dyed pink hair now showing roots.

'How can I help?' Dr Glick asks.

Anton admits to having little interest in work or anything else for that matter. He also recently split with his boyfriend.

'I met up with him the other day and I thought I was moving on,' he volunteers. 'But then I realised it was like when you're sitting on a train at the platform. And you think you're moving but you realise it's actually the train next to you.'

Dr Glick nods, no time for analogies. 'And how do you feel? Are you sleeping? Are you enjoying anything?'

'I feel shit . . . I can't sleep . . . and no, I'm not.'

'Eating?' Dr Glick asks.

'Not really. Although I have thought about downing a litre of bleach. Not that I would, probably.'

'I see,' says Dr Glick, reaching for her prescription pad. 'Take these every day and come back in a fortnight. Ben will show you out.'

Once back in her room Dr Glick asks for my diagnosis as she types her notes.

Not all that long ago Anton's diagnosis would have been 'homosexuality' to be cured with aversion therapy or even chemical castration. Thankfully things have moved on since 1973 when it was removed from the *DSM*, but it's still a perturbing reminder that the words we use in psychiatry aren't exactly a hard science.

'Depressive disorder, probably moderate type,' I say.

'And why?'

'As there are two core symptoms and some biological symptoms. The hallmarks being pervasive low mood, poor sleep, poor concentration, loss of enjoyment, loss of appetite and some suicidal thoughts with a considered method. All of which has lasted for more than two weeks,' I regurgitate, fresh from my textbook.

'And your treatment?'

'An SSRI, like the fluoxetine 20 mg you prescribed.'

'And if there's no improvement after two to four weeks?'

'Increase the dose. And if no improvement on maximum dose try a different class of antidepressant or augment with mirtazapine or venlafaxine as per the guidelines.'

'Good,' she says. It's a rare compliment from my boss and I feel proud that I'm slowly getting the hang of psychiatry.

Part of me does wonder if Anton's brain is really defective or whether he's simply experiencing the natural ups and downs of love. This certainly seems to be how Shakespeare described it in GCSE English, or did Romeo and Juliet also have undiagnosed severe depression (F32.2)?

'Um, Dr Glick?' I begin.

She pushes her keyboard away and looks up at me. 'Yes?'

But at that moment the receptionist pokes her head through the door again. Our 'three o'clock' is waiting.

Life is complicated enough sometimes. 'Never mind,' I say. Then I go to collect our next patient.

Two Fridays later, when the ward is surprisingly quiet, I seize the chance to shadow Dr Glick again in clinic. This time Anton's head is raised in the waiting room and when he catches my eye he springs up from his chair.

'How are you Anton?' asks Dr Glick inside her consultation room, pen in hand.

'I'm fine now. Feeling much better thanks. Sleeping . . . eating again. Thinking much more positively.'

'Any thoughts about drinking bleach?'

He laughs, shaking his head at the hilarity of his two-weeks-ago-self. 'I actually poured that stuff down the drain.'

'Excellent,' says Dr Glick. She catches my eye and I feel like we're sharing the victory. Although clearly the medicine has done most of the heavy lifting.

'Well I don't see any further role for us here. Let's discharge you back to your GP. I'll ask them to just keep doing what we're doing.'

As I walk our happy customer back down the corridor, I thank him for letting me observe his consultation.

'I've learnt so much. And it's great that the SSRI worked so well for you,' I gush.

'The what?'

'Sorry, the antidepressant. The one Dr Glick prescribed.'

Perhaps Anton confides in me because we're a similar age, or maybe it's a man-to-man thing or because he wasn't really given the chance on Dr Glick's clinic conveyer belt.

'Oh, I never took those,' he says sheepishly.

'What? But you seem so . . . different?'

'It's probably because I got back with my ex,' he says with a grin. He exits through the large glass doors where he's reunited with his boyfriend outside who's smoking a roll-up.

As I watch them walk off hand in hand I think of that Voltaire quote I never really understood: 'The art of medicine consists in amusing the patient while nature cures the disease.'*

Back in her office Dr Glick is typing the discharge letter to the

---

* Many mental illnesses are said to be 'relapsing and remitting' in nature, which means that they come and go. 'Statistical regression to the mean' is the idea that patients with some abnormality will, on average, tend to spontaneously improve anyway. For example, Posternak found that 85% of major depression cleared within a year even without treatment. Thus if a medicine is introduced during this time (presuming it's taken) one could wrongly conclude that the treatment caused the effect. It's a bit like how the Mayans performed human sacrifices to please the gods, not realising that the sun would have risen even if they hadn't ripped out poor Aapo's beating heart.

GP. 'Ben, describe fluoxetine's mechanism of action in Anton's brain?'

'Um, actually . . .' I begin. At this her face drops. Is it apprehension I can see, that perhaps the case isn't quite as simple as we've packaged it?

I don't want to rock the boat, plus I need Dr Glick to sign me off as fit to progress to the next year of training. Anton is better, why is immaterial I suppose.

'His improvement in mood is likely mediated by increasing the intra-synaptic levels of monoamines, primarily affecting 5-hydroxytryptymine,' I say, which definitely sounds better than 'got back with boyfriend'.

'Excellent Dr Waterhouse,' she says, certainty restored. 'You're starting to sound like a proper psychiatrist.'

As I cycle home, a backlog of thoughts catch up with me.

I remember how when at medical school I told a professor of cardiology I wanted to be a psychiatrist, he said 'You want to be a social worker with a stethoscope?'

Only now do I get what he meant. For many of the patients I've seen in my very short career their issues could be explained by problems of living just as much as any so-called mental illness.

For Anton it was his relationship break-up, but for others it's work stress, poverty, antisocial neighbours, crap housing, bereavement, loneliness, a lack of opportunity, purpose or hope, or the absence of any number of things that seem to be the necessary ingredients for a contented life.

Sometimes I wonder if the medical-sounding diagnoses, clusters and codes that I'm forced to enter on endless forms, couldn't more honestly be replaced by 'NFI' (no fucking idea), 'SLS' (shit-life syndrome) or 'PNA' (pretty normal actually). But without the time to explore people's lives, the impotency of a desecrated social care system to change them, or the ready availability of more thoughtful treatments, can I really blame overwhelmed GPs or psychiatrists for feeling like they need to 'do something' and writing an SSRI prescription which takes less than a minute?

I arrive home to a text from Nafisa. 'Are u still alive or has a patient killed u with a hot chocolate?'

Crap, I'd agreed to join some trainees in the pub after work. I text her an apology and promise to come to the next one.

'How r u anyway?' comes her reply.

I'm having a fundamental crisis of faith in my chosen speciality. Wondering if I've made an awful mistake. Paranoid that I'm just another 'barbaric' psychiatrist on the wrong side of history. And today's fresh concern; is psychiatry sometimes guilty of medicalising everyday life?

I look for the emoji which might best encompass all of this. But then I give up and just send her the flexed bicep one.

6

PEGGY

I'm not on-call this weekend so I've come up north to visit my paternal grandmother Peggy who, contrary to what my mum often says, is definitely not dying. Much to my granny's disappointment.

'Where's Grandpa?' my granny asks me again.

I hesitate and look at the black and white photographs of her late husband in his navy medals. My grandpa had a fierce, old-school temper and could explode at any moment. It probably wasn't helped by fighting in the Second World War which he never talked about. Before he died, when we all went to visit him my mum would do her thing of swinging her arm around from the front seat of the car to lovingly squeeze our thighs. Then she'd say, 'Boys remember not to mention the war, holidays or gay people.' Our grandpa would punch us in the back of the head for something as innocuous as wearing a cap back to front. Once, aged five, on my first ever bicycle lesson, I failed to weave between some canes he'd assembled in the garden, so he hit me across the face with one of them. He had high expectations and a short fuse but he was big-hearted. He got an MBE for his voluntary work helping the local community, and he had been teaching me how to ride a bicycle after all. I think my dad inherited his practicality, and his physicality, from him.

I used to always remind my granny that Grandpa had passed away, but her dementia meant she'd just end up grieving twenty times a day, the twentieth just as painful as the first. Her sadness seemed as raw as Anton's had been, after he temporarily lost his partner. It seems unnecessarily cruel to remind her so I recently changed my approach.*

'I think he's just out getting some milk,' I say. Other times he'll be pottering around doing odd jobs, hanging out the washing, posting a letter.

'Oh he's a good man,' she says. Maybe love isn't overrated after all.

In some rare excitement recently she started choking and her well-meaning carers called an ambulance which blue-lighted her to hospital. My mum constantly thinks my granny is on the brink of death, but she seems to be indestructible.

She is sitting, as usual, in her wheelchair wrapped in blankets. Her post-stroke muscles contort her limbs into unnatural positions and she constantly shuffles her bottom trying to find the elusive comfortable position she's been seeking for the last twenty years.

'So what's your news?' she asks me for the umpteenth time.

I sip my tea from a chipped Royal Jubilee mug whose handle has been repaired with superglue. 'Not much to report. How are you after your hospital drama?'

'God sent me back down to earth to try harder. Only the good die young Benji,' she adds flashing me an impish smile.

'You're going to live forever then,' I dutifully reply.

I know almost word for word from my visits how our conversations will play out. She said that line after her last choking episode – strokes often paralyse your swallow as well as your limbs. They don't help memory much either.

---

* Unlike most things in psychiatry the aetiology (cause) and pathology (disease process) of Alzheimer's disease and vascular dementia is known. Their effects can be seen on head scans and on brain autopsies too. But sadly this knowledge doesn't make dementia any more treatable.

When I offer her another cup of tea she'll say, 'Make it a double whisky,' even though she's teetotal and at parties used to pour her wine into plant pots. Next, she'll ask if I've met anyone yet and when I say no, she'll joke, 'You're over the hill, no one will ever want you at twenty-four.' Then I'll tell her that nowadays people don't always marry the first person they meet aged eighteen. I won't mention that I've not been twenty-four for several years now. Next she'll ask me, 'So how's medicine?' When I remind her that I now specialise in psychiatry she'll say her line, 'How can you have any faith in that nonsense when your mum is the way she is?'

One small benefit of my granny having a stroke in her frontal cortex (the area of the brain that usually controls inhibition) is that thoughts she might previously have kept to herself, she no longer does.* To most people, 'losing their inhibitions' is dancing on a table in a Yates's wine bar, but for my granny it means telling people they've got fat. Or in my case, bald. She also now liberally dishes out family secrets. She was friends with my mum's parents, that's how my mum and dad became first loves aged fourteen, so knows her side of the family well. 'You know your mum first saw a psychiatrist when she was six? For sadness, I think. Things have never been good with her sister.'

Whenever I've previously raised this with my mum she's denied it and blamed it on my granny's dementia.

'It runs in the family,' my granny continues. 'Her grandmother died in a psychiatric hospital.'

---

* In 1848 the American railroad foreman Phineas Gage became 'the man who began neuroscience' when an iron rod accidentally plunged through his skull and came out the other side. He miraculously survived but having destroyed much of his frontal lobe his friends noted his personality had changed. This gave rise to the now accepted idea that different brain regions serve different functions (and presumably also gave rise to the use of hard hats).

Not even my mum denies this. Apparently her gregarious grandmother was incarcerated because psychiatrists considered her 'unmanageable' which culminated in her attacking someone with a walking stick. When I asked my mum why she'd never told me this before, she said, 'You didn't ask.'

If we had a family motto, that phrase 'You Didn't Ask' would be it. Probably in Latin, *'Non Postulasti'*, to stop people enquiring. You would never know any of our family secrets unless you probed directly. Presuming you received an honest answer, of course.

I turn back to my granny who keeps wriggling, still looking for that position. My dad's family haven't always been so quick to acknowledge mental illness on their side of the family, but still. Growing up, strange behaviour would see my family threaten 'to send you to St Nick's', the Victorian lunatic asylum turned modern-day psychiatric hospital in Newcastle. Just as some exasperated mothers would promise to put their head in the oven if you didn't finish your greens. Good, solid, northern parenting.

Not all of my family managed to stay on the right side of a psychiatric hospital's locked door. Next to the photo of my late grandpa is one of my dad as a boy with his younger brother on Embleton beach during the summer holidays. My eccentric uncle Thomas is, for some reason, still dressed in full school uniform. This practical joker was also an adventurer and once canoed from Dover to Calais with his friends. He later went to York University and in his twenties began working as an architect. Then one spring day, quite out of the blue, he tried to drive off a bridge believing he was being chased by torturers. Mercifully he survived the wreckage, but paramedics quickly suspected he wasn't 100% well mentally. He was sectioned and admitted to a psychiatric hospital. My grandpa refused to visit him during that first long incarceration of many, or even acknowledge his new diagnosis of schizophrenia, instead preferring to think Thomas had just 'had a bad day'. So my granny would visit alone. As would my dad, who went nearly every day during that first six-month admission.

Growing up we knew Uncle Thomas as a man of few words who sometimes played football with us and when sitting on the sofa always rolled his head around and around and around which I now know to be a side effect of his antipsychotics. We knew he'd also occasionally go back into hospital where they ran up to 460 volts of electricity into his brain.

Predictably at some point I know my granny will change the conversation, hold my gaze and say she hopes I'll put her out of her misery when she 'starts' to lose her faculties. I'll nervously laugh and say I can't, not least because I'd miss her too much. Then she'll say, 'If I were a dog, you would've put me down by now.' I still don't have a response for that one.

There's no cure for dementia and France's healthcare system no longer bothers funding anti-dementia drugs given they do so little. And all the world's oily fish and Sudokus won't save my granny now. Dementia only ever progresses and the patient and family are forced to watch this cruel cerebral shutdown.

Because of this I've sometimes daydreamed about helping my granny by sourcing the necessary cocktail of pills or even holding a pillow over her face. But even if I could bring myself to do it, not all of my family would thank me. Plus I'd end up in prison.*

But what about 'voluntary euthanasia' where you're merely an inactive bystander while nature takes its course? Say if I just

---

* Assisted dying is now a service offered through Dignitas, and Swissair slightly morbidly advertise flights to Switzerland for '£59 one-way'.

stood there after a chunk of meat went down the wrong way again and nestled in her windpipe?

Luckily it's not an ethical dilemma I'll likely ever have to worry about in reality. Not least because when Rita, her endlessly cheery Hungarian carer, comes through with my granny's roast dinner, it's been entirely pureed into a Sunday-lunch smoothie of green, beige and brown splodges.

'Rita does this now because I choked the other day you know?' she says.

'I do Granny.'

In the background the TV hums, a celebrity chef preparing meals my granny will never get to eat.

'But God sent me back down to earth to try a bit harder,' she continues. 'Only the good die young Benji.'

'You're going to live forever then.'

She smiles. 'So, have you got a girlfriend yet?'

7

JAMAL

'Is this what you sick fuckers call entertainment?' Jamal shouts, staring down the lens of the CCTV camera. He turns, lowers his trousers and pulls a moonie 'for the millions watching back home'. In reality, it's just myself and my colleagues who get an eyeful.

Jamal was admitted a few days ago believing he's in a reality television show, colloquially known as Truman delusion. Body cameras are worn by staff on some psychiatric wards to document any abuse that they experience and to protect patients from any heavy-handedness. But the blinking red lights and whirring cameras only fan the flames of Jamal's delusional belief that he's in the reality show *Big Brother*. This prompted him to recently attack a nurse and destroy her body cam.

When brains fail, psychiatry defers to brawn. The nurse had activated her panic alarm and dozens of nurses had rushed in to restrain Jamal, then he was dragged to the 'seclusion room'. Modern seclusion rooms have replaced the infamous 'padded cells' of the old asylums,* leaving a sparse, white-walled space that's designed to minimise overstimulation. They're reserved for patients who are thought to be particularly disturbed or dangerous. Or for when psychiatrists run out of any better ideas.

Depriving someone of their liberty and restricting them not

---

* Padded cells, along with physical restraints like straightjackets, were phased out from the 1950s with the advent of powerful psychotropic drugs which could effectively restrain agitated patients chemically.

just to a psychiatric hospital but to a small, single room with only a mattress and a toilet, is controversial. Therefore scrupulous and regular checks are required day and night like the one I'm doing now with Blessing and the emergency response team. These are usually the beefiest team members from other wards trained in physical restraint, recruited not so much for their soft skills as for their muscle. Plus me.

Dr Glick asked me to do this one while she's in clinic.

I take a deep breath, the biggest nurse flings open the door and we enter the seclusion room. What Jamal calls the 'Diary Room'. Under the circumstances, it's probably good that I've now lost my Geordie accent. The emergency response team form a semicircle around him with me just behind.

'Hi Jamal, I'm Benjamin, one of the doctors.'

'Yada yada yada. I want to speak to the director. I'm opting out. Just give me the papers I need to sign.'

'Jamal you're in a psychiatric hospital—'

'I know it's just a set. Not even madhouses would be as shitty as this.'

I manage to stifle a smile at this scathing review of what is one of the better psychiatric hospitals.

'I know it's bare in this room, but this *is* a psychiatric hospital.' Maybe I should mention the excellent staff parking.

'Yeah, yeah I know you're a fake doctor you just say whatever's in the script. They haven't even got decent actors. Shit production. Shit script. Shit actors.'

Being told you do a bad impression of a psychiatrist certainly doesn't ease any sense of impostor syndrome.

Clawing for some legitimacy I show Jamal my ID badge, the one I was given at my induction eight months ago.

'That's a fake. It doesn't even look like you, that person isn't even that bald.'

I blush and look to Blessing, Omar and the others. Their facial muscles are working overtime not to laugh.

'Um, Jamal, we've er brought your medicine,' I stutter.

'I'm not taking those dummy pills. They're not even the right colour.'

Blessing stares at me, a silent reminder to tell him about the other option.

'If you won't take the tablets unfortunately we'll have to give you the injection.'

Jamal looks at the army of nurses. Then at their body cams, recording everything in high definition. Then to the now familiar-looking kidney dish holding a syringe-full of medicine or a paper cup of tablets.

I'm not sure which is more distressing to witness: restraining a patient and forcibly injecting them, or when after seventy-two hours in seclusion, now worn-down and wise to how things usually pan out, they just bend over and take it. Jamal reluctantly drops his kegs to reveal the bare cheeks of a bottom we're becoming quite familiar with. He winces as the needle pierces his skin, then he drops on to the mattress.

'Thanks Jamal. Do you have any questions for us?'

'What's the point?' he says woozily now, 'Everyone in here just lies.'

'Try me,' I say. 'I promise I won't.'

He slowly brushes a dreadlock out of his face. 'Well if this isn't a game show, what fucked-up social experiment is going on here?'

'How do you mean?'

'These medical studies you white doctors are doing on us black guys in here. Injecting us all with this stuff, I dunno what it is, pigment lightener or chemicals so we can't have babies?'

'That's honestly not happening Jamal. Its antipsychotic medicine to help you think more clearly. It's nothing to do with race.'

'So why are most of the people on this ward black? The patients, the cleaners, the caterers, these lot,' he says, flicking a floppy wrist at Blessing, Omar and the emergency response team. 'And every single doctor I've seen, like you and that Dr Glick, is white.'

The health inequalities which exist between genders, occur in relation to race too. Sometimes it takes those who are unwell to say what many sane people daren't acknowledge. First my receding hairline, and now this. Jamal is full of uncomfortable truths today.

I feel my face flush again. But this time the emotion is deeper, more shame than embarrassment. Now I don't look to the team for support. This time, I sense no one is smiling.

The psychiatric profession has a grim track record when it comes to race: from German psychiatrists colluding with Nazi eugenics programmes, to pathologising civil rights protesters as 'mad'. In the 1800s attempts were even made to label freedom-seeking black slaves with a mental illness called 'draepotomania' which supposedly explained their strange desire to try and flee their masters.

Even in modern times black men disproportionately fill up psychiatric hospitals, being four times more likely to be sectioned and ten times more likely to be diagnosed with psychosis.[1] They're also more likely than their white counterparts to be physically restrained, put in seclusion, admitted to Psychiatric Intensive Care Units (PICU), treated aggressively with drugs and to die in hospital.

This high prevalence of psychosis isn't replicated in Africa or the Caribbean, suggesting it isn't biological. It's no longer thought to be related to lifestyle either, since statistics suggest that white and black men smoke roughly the same amount of cannabis (skunk especially can increase the risk of psychosis). Is it because the black community seek help less due to a mistrust of public services given historical scandals against them, so when they do come into contact with services, they're more unwell and require more aggressive treatment? Or could societal discrimination in the form of racism, just like other traumatic life events, effect-ively *cause* schizophrenia? Or perhaps most troublingly for me, could it be that psychiatrists unconsciously give the grimmest diagnoses to black men and have a lower threshold for section-ing and forcibly medicating them due to ingrained ideas about their 'dangerousness' to society?*

'I'm disappointed in you brothers,' Jamal says to the emer-gency response team. The sedatives are kicking in and a string of drool falls from his mouth to the mattress. 'We're just slaves without chains in here.'

I'm trying to be less defensive during conversations about race. I can't pretend to be colour blind when I notice being the only Caucasian in a seclusion review or staff huddle, the white ele-phant in the room. It would be odd if I didn't notice, as someone brought up in a remote field in the north-east, the least ethni-cally diverse region of England. In our local village shop I once found Edam cheese in the 'exotic foods' section.

'I agree Jamal, there are some troubling ethnic differences between the patients and even the doctors and other hospital

---

* In 2018 an independent review of the Mental Health Act looked to under-stand numerous racial differences (a regrettably named parliamentary 'White Paper'). Amongst other things, it recommended improved representation of Afro-Caribbean staff at senior levels and attempting to correct decision-making bias. Several years on, though, things don't look much different.

staff here. But we probably can't fix these wider societal problems today. Also, just to say, if a white patient had attacked a staff member and destroyed their body cam, I'm pretty sure they'd be in seclusion too. So I don't think on this occasion it's to do with racism.'

'I hope you're right,' he says.

As part of my ongoing attempts to be more sociable with members of my trainee group, after work I go to Beatrice's flat-warming party. On the front steps some effortlessly cool people are smoking spliffs, so to seem more fun, before entering I untuck my work shirt.

Nafisa is throwing shapes in the living room, belting out the chorus of Beyoncé's 'Single Ladies (Put a Ring On It)', and waves at me.

'Hello stranger, you made it!' she says. I mime needing to put my corner-shop beers in the fridge and head to the kitchen. 'Try to have a good time! Go with the flow! Just imagine you're somebody else!' she shouts after me.

I generally try to avoid noise and crowds, but when I do brave a party I'll usually hide in the kitchen, my toes curled up inside my shoes and clenching my beer like a stress ball. Maybe it's a side effect of living in the middle of nowhere, failing to mix with anyone who wasn't a brother. Or maybe as my mum sometimes jokes, I have autistic spectrum disorder F84.0. Or maybe its OK to just say that I'm socially awkward and leave it at that.

As the music rattles the single-pane windows, I can't help thinking about the poor neighbours. 'It's quite loud isn't it?' I say to a girl leaning against the kitchen worktop. She's holding a can of Strongbow in one hand and trying to key some mysterious white powder from a baggie with the other.

'What?'

'It's quite loud!'

'It's a party,' she says looking around in search of better company.

Her face glitter is already smudged. She manages to get most of the substance up her nose, then balances some more on the end of the key and offers it to me.

'It's ket,' she says.

I'd much rather have a cup of tea but I've been told off before for boiling the kettle at parties. 'I'm good thanks,' I say, as if I've had an ample sufficiency of horse tranquilliser already today.

She shrugs and has my portion. 'So what's your thing?' she asks. 'You know, for work.'

Already in my short career I've had this in social situations where I tell people I'm a psychiatrist, they fear I can read their mind, so make an excuse to leave. Nafisa is always telling me to loosen up, try to have fun and to experiment with being someone else, and I guess I'll never see this woman again. I take a swig of lager for inspiration then let the first made-up job tumble from my mouth. 'Soldier,' I say.

'Oh, *really?*'

No one is more surprised by my answer than me. My family are Quakers, who are famously pacifists.

'Yeah I've just come back from . . . Afghanistan.'

'Wow. What's it like there?'

'Dusty.'

She nods enthusiastically. The less I say, the more she hangs on my every word. Traumatised war hero sort of vibes.

'Can I ask you, um, quite a personal question?'

'Anything,' I say generously. I'm getting quite into this. Maybe I can be fun after all.

'So, um, have you killed a lot of people then?'

I consider for a moment, what is a good answer for a soldier?

More is almost definitely preferable. It's probably no coincidence that my brain threw me 'soldier' as my fantasy job. The total opposite to medicine, where a high body count would usually raise eyebrows.

She's still looking at me expectantly.

I don't want to say too many or too few, so I keep it vague.

'Hard to say.'

She nods, respectfully, knowing not to push me. But I can't help myself.

'But probably . . . thousands,' I add.

Her face drops. Thousands is definitely too many. She leaves abruptly, probably even quicker than if I'd told her I was a psychiatrist.

I'm eyeing up the kettle when another of Beatrice's friends introduces herself as Claire. We get talking and she comments on my fading accent. When I tell her I'm originally from New-castle she slurs what a crazy coincidence it is as she went on a hen do there three years ago. Over her shoulder I can see Nafisa at the fridge getting herself another J2O. She clocks Claire, gives me a wink and does exaggerated thumbs-up at me, before return-ing to the dance floor. Clare tells me she's a fashion designer and inevitably asks me what I 'do'. I've had quite enough fun for one day so I come clean about being a psychiatrist.

'Oh, you don't want to get stuck with me. I'm mad me,' she says.

I think of Jamal in seclusion. It seems unjust that people like him rarely get airtime in the 'mental health conversation' which is generally dominated by high-functioning people with far milder issues or even armchair self-diagnoses.

Part of me wants to say to Claire, 'Oh yeah, do you think you're the queen of Egypt? Or do you scrawl messages on walls in your own menstrual blood? Or do you pull out your own teeth because you believe MI5 have bugged your fillings?'

But I just smile politely and say, 'Oh yeah, how come?'

She tells me she has ADHD but just 'undiagnosed'. She is beaming, with a proud smile on her face like she's won an all-expenses-paid holiday to the Caribbean. What's the etiquette here, am I supposed to congratulate her? I refuse to throw my arms around her and tell her it's brilliant news. I know some people find the contestable diagnoses we use helpful, but it seems perverse somehow when they start to become fashion accessories.

I ask what sort of problems she experiences.

'Oh, I'm always on my phone. And I always have like twenty tabs open on my Internet browser. And I struggle to focus on really boring tasks.'

I sometimes can't help feeling that through the noble aim of raising 'awareness', the challenges of everyday life have somehow been lumped in as 'mental illness'. I understand the seduction of having one of the now 400-plus medical-sounding labels from the *DSM* to pathologise and legitimise undesired behaviours, feelings or personality traits, but it does water down the experiences of people who are genuinely disabled by serious mental illness. People like Jamal who spend weeks, months, years and in some cases decades incarcerated in psychiatric hospitals unbeknown to most of society.

Or maybe this is just the cold, hardened mindset I'm already developing as a firefighting NHS psychiatrist who is forced to triage and only has the mental reserve for the most severe cases. Like how you'd struggle to hold an A&E doctor's attention for long telling them about your bunions. It would hardly matter if there were enough psychiatrists and adequate mental health resources to share around. But there aren't.

'I mean, I do all of those things,' I say.

'You should get yourself tested,' she says.

Out of curiosity I recently did an online screening tool and was surprised to be told I had 'symptoms consistent with ADHD' and to 'seek medical advice'. I am often distractible, restless and sometimes even impulsive but I feel like that's less a symptom of a brain disease and more a consequence of living in the twenty-first-century digital world where our attention is the commodity that tech companies are fighting for.

'But isn't all that stuff kind of . . . normal?' I gently push back.

She's standing perfectly still and isn't restless. She's also turn-taking during the conversation without interruption. God, I'm fidgeting more than her and I really don't think I have ADHD. The only remotely alarming thing is that she's wearing a fedora indoors.

She shakes her hand at me dismissively and changes the conversation. 'OK here's one Dr Psychiatrist, what's the secret to happiness?'

This is another commonly asked question. Another where we like to reduce life's complexity into a nice bite-size explanation.

'It's really very simple,' I want to say, 'all you need is a healthy birth, secure attachment, happy childhood, minimal or no trauma, high resilience to stress, loving friends, family and partner, fulfilling work, financial security, manageable targets, eight hours' sleep a night, regular exercise, healthy diet, access to nature, limited use of alcohol, drugs and social media, faith or spirituality, an acceptance of failure and death, an ability to process grief, a naturally positive outlook, maybe a pet, a gratitude journal, plus or minus antidepressants, therapy and 100% charge on your phone.'

But I just take a long sip of my beer.

'I think it's inflammation,' she says. 'I read it in an article. Depression is all just about gut microbes.'

It's good to know that in 2030 when depression becomes the

single biggest burden of illness in the Western world, we can cure it with industrial quantities of Yakult.

Later as I'm unlocking my bike the girl with the smudged face glitter from before, smoking on the front steps, says goodbye to me with a solemn salute.

8

GRAHAM

People find Jesus at different times in their lives. For Paul the Apostle it was on the road to Damascus. For St Augustine, it was after hearing a child's voice urge him to 'take up and read'. For those attending the 3–4 p.m. senior aqua aerobics class at the Get Fit Leisure Centre, it was when he tried to walk on water in the swimming pool's deep end and needed saving by the lifeguard.

When he said he was the son of God they sensed he needed more than just swimming lessons, and called an ambulance. He was taken to A&E, assessed and brought to Daffodil Ward where he's now sitting in a white hospital-issue dressing gown while his clothes dry.

He's arrived at a godawful time too, just after 6 p.m. as I was trying to make my escape to meet my brothers because Josh has had a painting selected for the BP Portrait Award. Josh has just texted me: am I still coming to the private view? Sipping wine and nodding at art feels another world away. I reply that I'll be there after I've dealt with the Second Coming and can get away from work, which he knows by now is a 'no'.

In the staff office Blessing runs me through the background and hands me a scrap of paper with his name, NHS number and date of birth, which I note isn't 25/12/0000.

You shouldn't judge people by appearances, but in psychiatry in the absence of any objective tests, we're forced to go into our mind palaces and detect subtle clues.

'So, he's the one in the . . . ?' I say, peering into the living area.

'The barefoot one in the white robe with long hair, yeah.

Incredible work Sherlock,' says Blessing. She raises her head from the night rota that she's trying to plug gaps in. 'If he's up for doing any miracles could you get me some extra staff for tonight?'

I exit the office and he gestures for me to approach, like one of the masses to be healed. I don't want to reinforce his grandiose delusion that he's the son of God so I just use the official name on his records. His Christian name.

'Hello Graham,' I say. 'I'm Benjamin, the ward doctor here.'

'I know who you are, my child.'

'Do you mind if I write a few things down?' I say, indicating my notepad.

His looks at me with kind, hazel-brown eyes. 'You wish to document my Gospel?'

'Um, not exactly. I just don't want to misquote you. And I would like to share what you tell me with my team if that's OK?'

'Of course,' he says smiling, proud that I'm spreading his words. 'Tell them the good news that Jesus of Nazareth, the King of Kings, has risen to save their souls.'

'OK, I'll certainly pass that on,' I say scribbling frantically to transcribe his phrases verbatim.

When I look up, he's taking in his new living space. 'What do you think I should do?' he wonders.

'Well, I think you need to be in hospital right now.'

'Yes you're probably right,' he says with a deep sigh.

Well, that was surprisingly easy. Perhaps he has a glimmer of insight into his illness after all?*

'I must stay here and heal the sick,' he adds.

---

* 'Insight' is the word used to describe a patient's ability to understand their illness. But it's also arguably just the word for when patients agree with the diagnosis that their psychiatrist gives them.

It dawns on me now that the one reason Graham isn't more angry is that he thinks he's here in a professional capacity. Maybe he heard Blessing's prayers for more staff.

'I will help however I can,' he says humbly.

I suspect that Graham is having a relapse of his bipolar affective disorder, and experiencing so-called grandiose delusions.

The psychoanalytic school of thought believes that psychosis is a natural defence from an unbearable reality. That transforming into an all-powerful, healing Jesus, literally God's right-hand man, helps Graham escape from his day-to-day mundanity as a forgotten member of society. And provides him with the father figure he's never had. It's an interesting formulation that could be explored with a psychologist. But even if we had one on our ward, psychotherapy sadly isn't thought to be much help for florid psychosis anyway.*

The more prevailing model in modern Western psychiatry is now that of brain defects and chemical imbalances. This is the only language that Dr Glick speaks. The tongue of 'proper doctors'. My prescription pad still sits in my bag, ready for my next placement. She lets me write drugs up on our inpatients hospital drug cards now too.

'How would you feel about taking a medicine?'

'What's it for, like a multivitamin or something?'

It's tempting to say, 'Yeah, it's just a multivitamin,' and get the

---

* In the 1960s the psychologist Milton Rokeach put three delusional men who all believed they were the Son of God in a therapy room together. He hoped that once confronted with each other's conflicting claims, they would be cured. It didn't work; they either believed the other men were mad or machines and even fought physically, which was slightly off-brand. Afterwards the humbled psychologist noted 'while I had failed to cure the Three Christs of their God-like delusions, they had succeeded in curing me of mine – of my God-like delusion that I could cure them'.

antipsychotic into Graham's body that way, but I vaguely remember that lying is one of those 'thou shalt nots'. Or to simply lace the ward porridge with olanzapine, Dr Glick's antipsychotic of choice, and give everyone a few dollops. Just as when I had a temperature, my dad would crush up the chalky paracetamol I struggled to swallow, and hide it in jam sandwiches. But nowadays autonomy is promoted over the paternalism of the past, so giving medicines covertly is less in vogue.

'Not exactly. It would be an antipsychotic called olanzapine, but a bit like a multivitamin it's supposed to make you well.'

'I must be strong for my mission, so I will take it.'

Before he changes his mind I write him up in a fresh medication chart for olanzapine 20 mg to be taken at night.

When I look back up Graham is leafing through a King James Version bound in blue leather that must've been in his dressing-gown pocket. Just as in hotel rooms, Bibles are usually kept on the ward which, along with a few Jeffrey Archers and P. D. Jameses, make up the patients' 'library'.

'Benjamin is a good Hebrew name,' he says, tapping the good book. 'The thirteenth child of Jacob.' He looks at me solemnly. 'Benjamin, do you believe?'

I don't think I do, and I've not even been baptised. Although after our village school failed its Ofsted inspection my mum successfully fought to get me and my brothers into the Catholic school in town, despite us not living in the catchment area. Or being Catholic.

Dr Glick usually deflects such personal questions with a textbook 'This isn't about me' or a 'Let's get back to the psychiatric interview'. But I sometimes think it can't hurt to give something, to try and even out the power imbalance, which if Graham hasn't detected yet, he soon will when he refuses medicine or tries to leave the locked ward. I remember how lucky I am to have the freedom to come and go and do nice things outside. At least in theory. 'I'm on the fence, agnostic,' I say, but this still feels like a measly offering. 'Although I am envious of my friend Nafisa who believes that God is always watching over all her decisions at work and—'

He interrupts me. '*Nafisa*? Which God?'

I tell him her God is Allah. He stands, his chair screeching against the linoleum floor.

'No no no no,' he's saying now while shaking his head. 'Benjamin you need to choose the right God.' There's a worrying zeal in his voice. 'Hellfire is hot brother!' he shouts, waggling his finger close to my nose, 'Hellfire is very hot!'

Maybe this is why doctors generally avoid getting into these sorts of things.

'Graham this isn't really about me,' I say. 'Should we get back to the psychiatric interview?'

I exit the hospital's main entrance probably around the time the wine glasses are being stacked in the art gallery's dishwasher. I ring Josh to apologise but he cancels my call.

I unlock my bike and cycle home through the darkness, now more aware than usual of the church, synagogue and mosque that I pass every day, dedicated worshippers queuing outside for evening prayer. As I pedal I wonder about the difference between people who think they're God's children, and Graham who believes he's the Son of God. Is believing that eating the body and drinking the blood of a 2,000-year-old Palestinian Jew every Sunday a form of madness? In his book *The God Delusion*, the evolutionary biologist and atheist Richard Dawkins certainly likens religion to a sort of mental illness.

I wouldn't go that far though. Faith, for people like my granny, serves her well. It gives her community and friends. I suppose it moves into mental-illness territory when the belief isn't widely held within a culture and endangers the person or others. Like if you nearly drown in the local swimming baths trying to walk on water.

Also, God could even be real. Although given the prevalence of false prophets I wonder if Christ ever did return to save humankind from climate catastrophe or nuclear war how long it would be before we banged him up in a psychiatric hospital?

The next morning Brian the bed manager enters the team office just as Omar is beginning our morning meeting.

'Sorry I'm late,' he says, perching on a work surface. 'Police outside have brought someone in the cage and won't go until we accept him. Any free beds here?'

Dr Glick shakes her head.

Brian takes his glasses off and massages his temples. 'OK lets go through the board and see.'

'Morning everyone,' Omar begins, standing beside the white-board of names. 'OK so yesterday evening we had a new admission, in Bed 3, I think Benjamin assessed him?'

I clear my throat. 'So for those who don't know, Graham Jones is a gentleman in his thirties with grandiose delusions that he's Jesus Christ who was brought into hosp—'

'We've not had a Jesus for a while,' interrupts Brian. 'Have you ever noticed they're always messiahs or billionaires or world leaders, they're never bin men or traffic wardens?'

I wince at his use of the word 'they' but I don't say anything. Dr Glick doesn't dignify his glib comment with eye contact, directing her response to the whiteboard. 'I think if you're going to have grandiose delusions, Brian, you probably aim a little higher on the pay scale. If it's not exceptional, well then it's just a delusion of mediocrity isn't it.'

That shuts Brian up.

'I prescribed him olanzapine 20 mg last night,' I say.

'Good idea Ben,' says Dr Glick, even though it's essentially what we do for everyone. 'Get something in his system early. Did he take it?'

Omar finds a squiggled signature on his drug card. 'He did.'

Brian senses an opportunity. 'If he's calm and compliant with meds then does he really need to be here? What's his risk of suicide?'

'Low, I think. He says he's only just risen from the dead to come and save us all so . . .'

'Risk to others?' he says.

'No, he's pretty peaceful and calm, generally. He is vulnerable to accidents though. For example, yesterday he nearly drowned trying to walk on—'

'Which one is he?' Brian says, cutting me off and peering into the living area. 'Oh, stupid question, bloke in the robe I'm guessing.'

Graham's clothes and shoes must surely be dry by now but he seems quite attached to his fluffy white dressing gown. And he's still barefoot.

'Well, he seems very settled,' Brian declares after less than five seconds. 'Medication is obviously doing the trick. If he's taking meds and risks are low, let's discharge him home or to a Crisis House. Least-restrictive practice and all. Then we can give his bed to the bloke in the cage.' He takes out his ringing phone, and cancels it. 'That's them calling now.'

'Least-restrictive practice' is the ethos, post-asylums and de-institutionalisation, of trying to treat patients in the community wherever possible. It's a noble aim, but I'm noticing professionals often hide behind this mantra as an excuse to kick people out of hospital before they're really ready.

'He looks better doesn't he Dr Glick?' says Brian, who is seeing Graham for only the first time.

'Um, he does seem a bit better,' Dr Glick says uncertainly. We watch as with flicks of water from a plastic cup, Graham tries to baptise the patients watching *Homes Under the Hammer*.

I agree to prepare his discharge papers.

Omar continues the board round. 'And in Bed 7, your friend is back Benjamin. Problem with her boyfriend again. Apparently, he's bashed in her front door.'

'Can I leave Paige with you?' Dr Glick asks.

I know by now that this is code for 'kick her out'.

'Um, sure. But what about her front door?'

'Not our problem,' says Brian. 'Tell her to call the police or the council.'

I doubt Paige would call the police, and I've heard other patients say it takes months for the council to address leaks, pests or mould. That's presuming they're not ignored completely.

I'm left with an increasingly familiar feeling of hopelessness.

'But, um, if we discharge her home, to the same living situation that brought her here, won't she just bounce back in a week or two?'

'Maybe,' says Dr Glick, impatiently, 'but she might not come here.'

My feeble protest over, the meeting continues. Afterwards I sit at a free computer, log in and try to read about Paige as Barbara and other disgruntled patients incessantly bang on the aquarium-thick glass. The buzzer goes from outside, Blessing answers it then replaces the intercom's handset.

'Benjamin I've got an early Christmas present for you. The police have now done all the paperwork and brought up the guy from the van.'

'Oh, right. Thanks.'

An angry, seemingly intoxicated man enters the ward in hand-cuffs with police. Having now seen hundreds of patients I've acquired a gut feeling about the presence of true mental illness, and this bloke seems more like an antisocial drunk who's somehow blagged his way on to a psychiatric ward. I direct them into a free consultation room with the guy still hurling abuse. A policeman hands me the patient's papers which I sign to say we've 'received' him, as you would an Amazon delivery. But unfortunately not the sort you can just leave with a neighbour.

'And um, I'll be needing those,' the policeman says, looking at the handcuffs. 'Am I OK to take them off?'

'I dunno, why did you put them on him?' I ask.

'He was beating up a load of our officers.'

This man should really have gone to the Psychiatric Intensive Care Unit (PICU), but they likely don't have any free beds.

I look at the six beefy police officers dressed in riot gear who were required to overpower him. Then at the female student nurse in a plastic apron who has come along as my backup. I haven't even stretched my hamstrings yet.

'Best leave them on.'

'Chips? Need 2 talk 2 u' says the message from Nafisa, then when I don't answer within an hour: 'It's important.'

Inside the canteen she's sitting at a window table with two large plates of our favourite golden, deep-fried sustenance.

'Benj I've really messed up,' she says, not even a hello.

She tells me that because her consultant is away she's been running the ward. Which happens. There should be a registrar, someone who's between us and our consultants in seniority, but there just aren't enough psychiatrists.

She tells me a patient was admitted with depression following an overdose.

'He seemed brighter, and he'd started reading again,' she says. 'The nurses said so too. He asked if he could get off the ward to read in the park. It was a nice day and he seemed fine. Plus I was really busy so I said he could have thirty minutes of unescorted leave. We didn't have enough staff for an escort, obviously.' She's crying now, tears salting her untouched chips. 'But he didn't go to the park, did he? He drowned himself in the fucking Thames.'

She sits up straight to compose herself, sniffs and rubs her nose with the back of her hand. 'Police identified him and also found the book he'd been reading. I didn't even have time to ask him what it was. It was *The Bell Jar* by Sylvia Plath.'

'Fuck,' I say, probably unhelpfully. My bedside manner is a work in progress. 'That's so sad. I don't think people can blame you though,' I try to reassure her, even though I'm not really sure about that at all.

Millions of people have read Sylvia Plath and don't go and put their head in an oven afterwards. But I'm quietly wondering if in the inevitable investigation into what happened, people will discount the understaffing and the fact Nafisa was forced into a level of responsibility she's not trained for and scapegoat her as a bad psychiatrist. Statistically, being a 'foreign doctor' probably won't work in her favour either.[1]

'He was getting better too. He had more energy. I should've known that's a risky period,' Nafisa continues.*

It crosses my mind that next year when working in the community, after their thirty-minute clinic appointments with us,

---

* It requires some 'get up and go' to kill yourself, so psychiatrists must be mindful that when severely depressed patients improve, they can rediscover the energy to act on their suicidal thoughts. Psychiatrists should also worry about suicide when depressed patients deteriorate, or get stuck and don't move in either direction, which doesn't leave much room for peace of mind.

our patients will return to the real world effectively being on leave *all* the time and free to do whatever they please. I bury the thought.

'You know the most fucked-up thing?' Nafisa says. 'When Brian the bed manager heard what had happened, he called me and asked "So does that mean there's now a free bed on Tulip Ward?"'

9

JOSEPH

I'm standing outside a grand white house on a wide leafy street in North London with a festive wreath on the front door. I press the buzzer for Flat 7, take a deep breath and say my name into the intercom. A voiceless *click* allows me in, which makes sense. I've heard that psychoanalysts use their words sparingly. Considered silences from the start.

Psychiatrists are encouraged to have their own therapy but I've delayed coming until now. I'm absolutely certain it has nothing to do with what happened to Nafisa.

I'm greeted at the top of the stairs by a grey-haired gentleman in his late sixties wearing chinos, a brown cardigan and sensible shoes. 'Hi Benji, I'm Dr Moore,' he says with a warm smile, and we shake hands for what will be the only time I ever touch him. Once inside he shuts the front door and I follow him past a small waiting room and through two more doors into the treatment room.

'Shut the doors after you please,' he says.

I do as instructed, closing the outer and then the inner door, only one inch apart, as though installed by a cowboy builder who got their measurements wrong. I wonder why they're like that.

'They're good for soundproofing,' Dr Moore says, seemingly reading my mind. 'So people's unconscious minds remain private.'

'Less good for storming out dramatically, since there are two doors to slam,' I joke.

'It sounds like you're already planning your exit Benji.'

Dr Moore lowers himself on to a chair at the head of a

buffed-up leather couch. *The* couch. Am I expected to do the introduction session horizontal? I hover momentarily as he observes me; his legs crossed, digits interlaced except for his two vertical index fingers which are to his lips and perfectly still.

'This is just the get-to-know-you session isn't it?' I say.

'That's right.'

'Ah good,' I say, heading towards the familiarity of a chair on the other side of the room. 'I thought for a second you wanted me on the couch.'

'I do,' he says. 'That's where we *really* get to know you.'

I look at the chesterfield couch with a pillow at the end like in Woody Allen films. Then I look back at the chair. Oh God, is where I sit going to *mean* something?

'Nice picture,' I say looking at the ambiguous print hanging on the wall in front of me. It's a Rorschach-like inkblot of blobs and blotches that looks exactly like blood-soaked roadkill.

'What do you see?' Dr Moore asks. He's now lowered his hands from his face and they're fanned and sitting in his lap, connected by the fingertips. In fact, Joseph's hands never seem to come apart, as though he's been involved in some sort of super-glue accident.

'Maybe a butterfly?'

He smiles knowingly. 'So Benji, how would you like to begin?'

'Um, well before we get started. I was wondering. Since you're calling me Benji, could I just call you Joseph?'

'Most people call me Dr Moore, you know, doctor–patient boundaries and all that—'

I interrupt him. 'Yeah I know but I'm not a patient. I'm just here for educational purposes,' I say, jamming my hands into my pockets casually as though we're colleagues chewing the fat.

'You are?'

'Yeah, for my training you know? Dr Glick said it would make me a better psychiatrist. So first names would be better. Less formal.'

Dr Moore peers at me over his glasses, which are low on his nose. 'OK why not. Therapy is an experimental space after all. And will you be standing up throughout all of our sessions too?'

It is a bit weird that I'm still standing. I turn around from the picture of the squashed badger. Then sit down in the chair.

'Lets start with some ground rules. So when we meet, which will be either four or five times a week—'

My mouth falls open. 'Pardon?!'

'Look Benji, this is just understandable resistance to meeting your unconscious mind.'

'Well Joseph my conscious mind is also resisting me being totally skint.'

'I always give a reduced rate for NHS workers. Say £50 for a fifty-minute session?'

The same cost as a premium sex line, or so I've been told. I feel like I'm bartering with a market trader selling gooseberries by the pound, rather than a professional therapist.

'OK, but I can only afford once a week. Besides I'm definitely not five-times-a-week messed up.'

Joseph considers. 'Fine, let's start with that. I'll be taking Christmas off, so let's start from January. So every week you'll come and see me, or rather my ceiling. Ideally you'll be on the couch.'

He gestures towards the upholstered piece of leather furniture next to him, as though perhaps I just haven't noticed it.

'And life is best understood backwards. So I'll sometimes ask you about your family, childhood, school, friends, traumas, sex, all that sort of thing.'

I nod. 'Right. So how do we know when I'm done?'

He laughs. 'You don't just wake up one day "cured". Analysis is an ongoing process of self-discovery. For some it's lifelong.'

Talking therapy that never ends sounds like a dud. Behind Joseph is a full bookcase with tomes of art and philosophy. Not much science.

'Why does it take so long though? Cognitive behavioural therapy only takes like six to eight sessions, doesn't it?'*

He chuckles. 'Yes but quick fixes don't generally last. It's just a sticking plaster like medicines. Popping pills may numb pain but it doesn't get to the root of problems. It's like taking paracetamol for toothache instead of extracting the rotten decay.'

I nod.

'Also, in here you don't have to be prim or proper, this is a safe space to experiment with being authentic. If you feel angry with me, be angry. Just no crossing of the physical barrier please.'

'Don't worry Joseph I'm not exactly the violent type.'

'Well no, and most people I see like you who've grown up around the things you have never go on to—'

'Like me?'

'The patient questionnaire you sent back?'

In amongst all the usual drama on Daffodil Ward I've completely forgotten that weeks ago to secure our initial appointment, I completed and sent back a new-patient questionnaire. I was urged to be as open as possible and a one-word or single-sentence answer wouldn't suffice in the large empty space by each question.

'Oh yeah. Um, about that, I presume everything's confidential?'

'Pretty much. Unless you tell me you're planning to murder someone. Then I'd be legally bound to tell the police.'

'Grass.'

---

* The NHS favours the time-limited and cheaper model of CBT which usually discharges people after about eight sessions. It teaches someone to think differently but isn't interested in *why* they think as they do.

He meets my flippancy with a blank expression. 'Benji I've noticed you like to use humour as a defence.'

'Sorry I think I'm just nervous.'

'Naturally. But you can't live your whole life making light of things to cover up pain. I've got some comedians on my books and they're some of my most depressed patients. Probably just below the psychiatrists.'

My eye is drawn to a box of tissues on a low table in front of him.

'I bet you get those in bulk from a cash and carry,' I say.

Joseph ignores this. He crosses his legs the other way and his trouser leg rides up to reveal colourful striped socks. Then he picks up some papers from the coffee table. 'A few things struck me about your questionnaire answers.' He licks his fingers before turning the pages. 'The first is that you're a trainee psychiatrist. The family bits, obviously. And the fact you left the relationship-history section blank.'

10

CHRISTMAS

'Tis the season to be jolly, unless you're an inpatient on a psychiatric ward. Or working on one. On Boxing Day morning, just before 8 a.m., as most of the country is still in bed or waking up to leftovers, I enter Nightingale with its familiar, clinical smell of antiseptic. A fake Christmas tree in reception has some sad-looking baubles, but no tinsel in case patients try to hang themselves with it.

My NHS trust sent personalised Christmas cards to our homes, which was a lovely touch. A clerical error meant they all had the wrong names inside, but I'll always treasure the card from my employers wishing 'Melinda' a happy Yuletide and thanking her for all her hard work.

For the first time in three years since becoming a doctor I wasn't on-call on Christmas Day so I spent yesterday with my family up north, a fleeting sixteen-hour visit.

'Can't you just explain that we're snowed in?' my mum said as I ate my breakfast cereal. She was sipping red wine as she cooked with the confidence of someone who knew that on Christmas morning, drinking was beyond criticism.

She had a point, to be fair. There'd been another huge dump of snow the previous night. The road gritters never come this far out which makes travel impossible. It would be a legitimate excuse for HR but they'd never find a replacement for me on Boxing Day.

My dad came in through the back door from defrosting the water pipe in his trademark jumper and jeans speckled with concrete and paint, held up by a makeshift twine belt. His hands are huge, calloused and swollen from a life of manual labour. At least one of his fingernails is usually black from a stray hammer blow. He's so strong he can carry a breeze block in each hand like light shopping. He wasn't wearing gloves, a hat or a coat, obviously.

'We'll find a way to get him there,' he said, overhearing our conversation.

My mum threw her hands up to her head. 'Oh John!'

My dad walked back outside into the blizzard, like an under-dressed Captain Oates. With his rusty red tractor we both cleared away the shin-deep snow carpeting the almost-vertical road which leads down to our secluded house which is sur-rounded by hills and trees. As we worked I could see my mum in her apron, watching us from the kitchen window, shaking her head and praying it couldn't be done.

Afterwards there was time for our customary happy but some-times tense family meal. I think because of my mum's work as a child psychologist she's seen the breakdown of the family unit lost to the TV dinner, so we've always eaten together, as if that is evidence enough that we are still a normal, functioning family. One of my brothers had laid the table, positioning the knives and forks perfectly straight, trying to make everything just right. My mum had decorated the table with a red cloth, sprigs of holly, and loads of candles. We always eat by candlelight, I think to try and create a calm atmosphere. We even have candles at breakfast.

As we ate our festive feast with everyone on their best behav-iour, my mum kept glancing out of the window, hoping that more snow would fall so she could keep all of her boys at home, but none did. I hugged her goodbye, then my brothers, then my dad did his white-knuckle snow driving, zigzagging up our steep hill. Then the car skidded and slid the other treacherous two miles down to the village, with my hands on the dashboard, and my dad telling me 'It's alright, it's alright.' We got there unscathed, as we always do, if you discount that he's written off two cars. From the village onwards, the gritters had turned the powdered snow to cola-coloured slush, and my dad drove me to Newcastle bus station for the Megabus back down to London.

So now, after a Herculean effort, here I am. Pulling my weight, one of the team, looking forward to standing shoulder to shoulder with my colleagues to cope with the Christmas onslaught.

'You're going need to cover both A&E and the wards today,' the night doctor tells me cheerfully. 'The other senior house officer can't make it – snowed in apparently. Happy Christmas, by the way.'

I cross over to the general hospital and follow a porter in a Santa hat into A&E.

My first patient here looks like the stereotypical 'cockney wrong 'un' in a Guy Ritchie film. Skinhead. Dubious facial scar. Millwall football shirt. And being handcuffed to the side rails of a hospital bed hardly waters down any look of criminality. Two policemen stand either side of him, trying to merge into the background by taking their hats off.

'Hi Damien, I'm the psychiatrist Dr Water—oooh can I get some help please!'

He's fitting. Staff rush in to help. Damien is wide-eyed, his arms and legs jerking violently, neck cocked back but it lasts less than thirty seconds. Luckily, he hasn't bitten his tongue or wet himself, as can sometimes happen.

He was brought here earlier today by police. He had been caught red-handed stealing a car radio but unfortunately for him had a seizure at that exact moment, thereby preventing a getaway. A&E can't find a cause for the fits which aren't brought on by flashing lights but seemingly by the sight of authority figures. Clinicians can increase a patient's blood pressure in 'white-coat hypertension'; is this its rare neurological sister? If authority figures are the trigger, I'm almost flattered. Two fingers to those people who say psychiatrists aren't 'proper doctors'.

Damien is also hearing voices. It's all very strange.

A medic in blue scrubs updates me. Damien's observations and physical examination were normal. His cranial and peripheral nerves were 'unextraordinary' (a good thing, in medicine you don't want to be 'extraordinary'). The results of a head scan and EEG, the gold standard for diagnosing epilepsy, will be back soon. 'But as you just saw, the fits are rather . . . atypical,' the medic says before exiting the cubicle.

'Hello again Damien,' I say after redrawing the paper curtains. 'Are you back with us?'

'Yeah.'

'Do you know where you are? Can you remember who I am and what day it is?'

'I didn't hit my head that hard. We're in hospital. You're the shrink. And it's Boxing Day.'

So he's not post-ictal, a confusion which sometimes follows an epileptic fit.

'That's right.' A glint of sunlight reflects off his handcuffs. 'I'm just trying to piece all this together. Can you tell me what happened earlier?'

Damien has complete amnesia of today's events. The police say he was stealing a car radio but that can't be right. He says he doesn't even watch TV after 10 p.m. because he doesn't like the foul language.

I ask about his personal history. Childhood was 'hard'; he was the youngest of eight, his mother was a part-time factory worker and his father was a full-time drug addict. Damien left school at fifteen, over some 'mix-up' involving joyriding. His girlfriend, a barmaid at his local pub, is expecting their first child.

'I wanna be a good dad, you know? Not like my old man,' he adds. On his phone he shows me a photo of the latest baby scan.

'Very nice,' I say smiling at the black and white blob on the ultrasound.

He has another look himself, smiles and returns the phone to his pocket.

Returning to business the police constables volunteer that they caught Damien down a cul-de-sac and shouted for him to stop. That's when he fitted.

The more junior officer, the one wearing plenty of Lynx deodorant, pipes up. 'I heard loud noises can do it. Maybe we triggered it by shouting?'

The doctor from earlier pokes his head through the flimsy curtains. 'Just to say, the CT head and EEG both came back normal too,' and then he's gone again.

'Well that's good news,' I say to Damien.

'What about the auditory hallucinations?' he says.

Use of medical jargon usually implies a medical professional or a layperson who's done their homework.

'What do you mean by "auditory hallucinations"?'

'The voices in my head.'

'Do they sound like they're talking inside your head or more like my voice does now?'

'. . . inside.'

Interesting.

Dr Glick has taught me that a crude way of distinguishing the origin of voices is by their location. More serious, schizophrenia-like voices are typically *external*. It's the voices *outside* your head that you really want to worry about.*

'What do they say?' I enquire.

'Um, they tell me to do things . . . stupid things like er . . . steal car radios. That's what they were saying earlier today anyway.'

I thought he couldn't remember anything about earlier.

'I couldn't see anything about hearing voices on your record,' I probe. 'Have you spoken to anyone about them before or is there a family history?'

'No.'

'And do you drink alcohol? Any beer, wine, spirits?'

'No! I've already been over all of this. How many more questions? I'm bursting for a piss.'

Over time Damien has become less comfortable talking, with beads of sweat collecting on his brow. When he held his phone up to me he was tremulous. Maybe this isn't psychosis but *neurosis*. Social anxiety perhaps?

'You go to the toilet Damien – I'll wait.'

'Do the rozzers have to come in with me again? It's degrading. I might need a crap.'

Damien's on '2:1 observations' so two people must always have eyes on him even during his most private moments. But

---

* In contrast, less serious pseudo-hallucinations found in our self-critical monologues, personality disorder, or intrusive OCD-like thoughts are usually heard *inside*. Relatively speaking, that voice in your head that dares you to push someone in front of the Tube, kick a cat or French-kiss your granny are *fine* – medically speaking anyway – you're having such thoughts because of your neurotic over-awareness of what *not* to do, and you almost certainly won't act on them. Fingers crossed.

maybe if I bend this rule for him, he'll open up. And I do sympathise, I can't even wee with someone at an adjacent urinal.

'OK, but you'll need to keep the door ajar.'

The older, balding officer unlocks Damien from the bedrail and reattaches him to his own wrist, like a briefcase full of money. We lead him to the single toilet cubicle, uncuff him and close the door but for the policeman's black boot between it and the doorframe.

'Are you OK in there?' I call, after a few minutes. No response. 'Damien?!'

Shit, maybe he's fitted? Or he's hanged himself from the light-switch cord? Or, maybe he's swum down the toilet U-bend and through the sewage works like in Shawshank *and is now at large nicking more car radios?*

We rush inside.

The good news is that Damien is alive. He's by the sink, his head cocked to the side and stooped underneath the hand dispenser, rhythmically pumping shots of the clear gel into his mouth.

He looks up at us, says 'Sorry,' and does a final few squirts for good measure. When he emerges he's forgotten to wash his hands but his oesophagus must be pristine. The older copper escorts Damien back to the bedside, less gently this time. The policeman with the bum-fluff chin does that finger-circling-around-the-temple-sign as if to say 'how crazy is *this* guy?'

I wonder if he thinks this is how psychiatrists communicate about patients. Maybe the more severe the illness, the bigger and more vigorous the finger's circular motion?

I sense he doesn't know that as well as killing 99.9% of germs, hospital hand sanitiser also contains 70% alcohol.

Damien hops into bed a new man. He's all smiles as he's handcuffed back to the side-rail and I notice his tremor has vanished. He's no longer withdrawing.

'Was that the aloe vera-flavoured one? It's quite nice actually,' he says cheerfully, as though offering tasting notes on a fine wine. The hand-soap sommelier.

Maybe it's my fault for focusing my checklist on drinks behind the bar, rather than industrial products underneath the sink.

'Right Damien, I'm glad you're feeling more um . . . comfortable. You were telling me about these voices you've been hearing. Could I call your girlfriend back just to see if she's noticed anything unusual?'

'No don't,' he says, a look of genuine concern spreading over his face. 'Stress can harm the baby.'

I give him a reassuring nod. 'And can you hear the voices now?'

'All the time, yeah.'

'But you can follow my voice. You're not distracted or preoccupied.'

At this Damien strikes his head with the palm of his hand, as though trying to dislodge water from his ear. 'Shut up!' he shouts into the room, then turning to me adds, 'I think I need to go to the madhouse.'

With this performance Damien would struggle to get into a village hall pantomime.

On Daffodil Ward I've learnt that in psychiatry the sickest patients, like Barbara, Jamal and Graham often lack the insight to realise that they're ill. So ironically asking for help, as people like Paige do, actually implies a reassuring degree of wellness. With constant bed shortages, psychiatric beds are reserved for only the sickest, and thus increasingly patients are admitted involuntarily under the Mental Health Act.[1] If you're a patient trying to get a psychiatric bed in the NHS, the worst thing to do is to ask nicely.

'Are you gonna admit him then, Doc?' says the first police-man. 'Because if you don't deem him to be mentally ill, he'll come back to the station with us. And he's breached his bail so he'll go back to the nick.'

'I didn't know he'd been in trouble before,' I say.

'He has,' the officer says with a certain world-weariness.

My hunch is that like Captain Blackadder, Damien is malingering; feigning symptoms to avoid an unwanted outcome. It's rare and not as easy as just putting some underpants on your head and pencils up your nose. But for psychiatrists, distinguishing fakery from insanity is also fraught with difficulty.*

I call the duty consultant for advice. One good thing about being junior is you can always hide behind a senior's decision. 'Sounds like barn-door malingering to me. He's trying it on. Discharge him and let the police take him away,' he says.†

The anonymous voice has the casual tone of someone advising me on how to repair a bicycle puncture. It must be easier to make decisions on faceless beings. To him Damien isn't an impish football fan, partner to Kelly or excited father-to-be.

I have a pang of guilt that when in trouble not everyone has a grandfather who can intervene and pay for them to go to a

---

* In a now infamous 1970s study called 'Being Sane in Insane places', actors presented at psychiatric hospitals claiming to hear voices. None actually had a mental illness, none were Hollywood-trained, yet all were admitted and diagnosed with schizophrenia except for the actor who attended a private hospital who was diagnosed with bipolar (because you get what you pay for). The trouble was that even after these healthy impostors stopped reporting voices and behaved entirely normally, they *still* couldn't get discharged from hospital.

† In the book *One Flew Over the Cuckoo's Nest* (written by former psychiatric hospital assistant Ken Kesey) and the later film starring Jack Nicholson, the criminal Randle McMurphy feigns mental illness to avoid imprisonment. But psychiatric hospital isn't as cushy as he imagined. Enforced shock therapy and a lobotomy render him a human vegetable (spoiler alert), so he might have been better off taking his chances with the rapists and murderers. At least in prison, you're given a release date.

decent school as mine did. Or the money to splash out on red wine at Christmas, rather than NHS hand-sanitiser.

'I just don't suppose prison will help Damien much either,' I say.

The consultant laughs. 'I agree it's pretty hopeless. But it just whiffs of antisocial behaviour with some alcoholism if you ask me. The "psychosis" sounds very suspicious. Medics weren't convinced by his fits either. Sounds like textbook trying-it-on more than true mental illness, so that's a problem for the criminal justice system, not for us.'

Chucking Damien in prison again, away from his partner and unborn child, feels a strange kind of justice. And not really in the spirit of Christmas.

'Alright,' I say flatly.

'Look, these are just some of the tough decisions you have to make, this is the job.' Before putting down the phone he reassures me, 'don't worry, you'll get used to it.'

I return to the bedside, wondering how to essentially call Damien a liar to his face. 'I've discussed your case with a senior colleague,' I begin. Damien is no longer distracted and looking directly into my eyes. 'I'm sure you'll agree there are some inconsistencies here. The fits, the voices, the alcohol gel. I understand why you're doing it, but I'm afraid you're not getting into psychiatric hospital today.'

I brace myself for an attack, either physical or verbal, but nothing comes. If only I could have police presence for *all* difficult conversations. He seems surprisingly relaxed about the prospect of thick-skinned porridge each morning, but I suppose he's done prison time before. Or, is Damien's ambivalence explained by a fog of undiagnosed psychosis?

The unsettling thing about psychiatry I'm discovering is that you can never be 100% certain about anything. Psychiatrists work in a constant cloud of grey. Occasionally brightened up by the psychedelic colours of madness. No two psychiatric presentations are ever the same. There are *thousands* of different combinations of symptoms that could qualify you for a diagnosis of depression. Damien's 'atypicality' is odd, but isn't oddness what we specialise in?

'So we can take him back to the station?' the second police officer says, and I nod. Thankfully he doesn't ask me if I'm sure.

They help Damien off the bed, recuff him to the bigger policeman's chubby wrist and make to exit through the curtains. As Damien passes me I scour his face for a final tell, a cheeky wink or a smirk to reassure me that my malingering hunch is right. I'd even take being spat on for some certainty. But no such luck and he's straight-faced as he's led away.

Meanwhile, outside hospital the country kills time before celebrating the turning of the year in that perfectly normal British way of getting absolutely battered.

11

LEON

A cruel thing about training as a doctor is that just at the point you start to settle into a job, you're moved on to another placement.

'Um, today is my last day here,' I announce after my final morning meeting on Daffodil Ward. 'So this is just a little something to say thank you.'

On our Sunday phone call my mum, a thoughtful gift-giver, suggested getting a plant and I liked the idea of living in the team's memory longer than the time it takes to eat a box of Celebrations.

So this morning before work I cycled via a florist. I wanted a mini lemon or lime tree, something fun and colourful to brighten up the office space. But the woman in 'Plantology' said their latest delivery was delayed so they didn't have much stock. The red roses were too romantic. The white lilies too sombre. It would just have to be one of the cacti. I chose the least lethal-looking one.

'Be careful with it,' I say, handing the gold gift bag to Dr Glick.

'Oh, wine maybe?' says Blessing hopefully.

Dr Glick peers inside, then slowly lifts my offering out by its pot. 'Thank you,' she says after slightly too long. She forces a smile but her lips look like they're being held up by strings.

'Well clearly that can't stay here!' Brian says, looking nervously over his shoulder.

He's a stickler for the often nonsensical rules and disapproves of my lunches here because he says it doesn't 'look good' having doctors eating out of the bins. I'd rather not fish it out of a black bag, and even floated the idea that staff join the patients in the dining room and eat what is left over. It would reduce food waste, give staff a boost with a free lunch and create less of a sense of 'them' and 'us' between patients and staff. But apparently that would be 'inappropriate' and a poor use of time. So instead, most staff spend fifteen minutes going to the canteen to buy an overpriced sandwich to eat alone in front of a computer.

'Why can't it stay here?' I ask, finding some final-day defiance.

'Oh, maybe just the fact that a patient could use it as weapon,' Brian says as though I've gifted the team a meat cleaver.

It's coming back to me, that even flowers are banned here at Nightingale Hospital. Barbara's brother visited from America bearing a bouquet. He came outside visiting hours, though, so was told he'd have to return the following day. Someone told Barbara that an unknown gentleman had delivered a bunch of flowers, which would have to be destroyed, presumably in case anyone had an allergic reaction to tulips. For twenty-four hours until her brother returned, Barbara thought they were from Harry Styles, which certainly didn't speed up her recovery.

I look again at the thick barbs, with ivory spines protruding from the dark green stem. Touching them would be like playing lucky dip inside a sharps bin.*

But being my last day, Dr Glick, seems willing to gloss over my ill-advised present. She clears her throat to say a few words. 'Ben I feel bad we haven't got you anything, so why don't you have this from us?' she says. And with that, she hands the cactus back to me.

At the end of the day I leave my keys in the office for the trainee replacing me tomorrow. Then I say goodbye to the staff and our current crop of patients.

---

* The plastic yellow bins for used needles.

When I worked as a junior doctor for two years in surgery and medicine I put on weight gorging on all the 'thank you' chocolates that were left lying around the wards by patients, but during my first year as a psychiatrist I've become fairly lean again.

My highlight of last week was when I told a sectioned patient he couldn't go home and he shouted, 'How does a baby-faced twat like you have the power to keep me here against my will?' It warmed my heart to be told that I still looked young.

I'm very touched that one patient, despite his florid psychosis, has got me a leaving present: a picture of a flower that he's drawn on a sheet of toilet paper. The GMC and BMA have strict rules on not accepting gifts from patients above the value of £50, but unless he's the next Van Gogh and this is a priceless original from his Daffodil years, I think I'm probably safe.

There's a sense of circularity as Blessing leads me out, back down the ward's long corridor with the bedrooms either side of us now occupied by new people. Over this year I've seen patients come and go. And then come back again, in the case of people like Paige. Graham was recently brought back to Daffodil Ward too because at the Crisis House he was trying to turn the contents of the water cooler into wine.

Most of the hundreds of patients who we've processed through the mental health machine, though – people like Anton, Barbara and Gladys – I will never see again, the next chapters of their stories a mystery.

I'm looking forward to working in the community where I will see less acutely unwell patients for up to a year. Some welcome time to get to know the person beneath the label.

Blessing and I enter the air lock together. In this strange place it hardly feels like twelve months have passed, time distorting just like some of our patients' realities.

Blessing releases me on to the other side and gives me a hug, being careful not to prickle herself on my cactus.

'Good luck Benjamin. Try not to miss us too much,' she says with a chuckle. 'I know how much you liked our food. And our parking.'

Then she clangs the doors shut behind her, a hard full stop to my year on Daffodil Ward, and I'm back once again in the free world.

Later that evening I meet Nafisa to celebrate making it through our first placements as psychiatrists.

'We survived!' I say, chinking my pint against her soft drink.

'Well, not all of us.'

'Oh shit. Sorry Nafs. That really wasn't your fault you know?'

'I didn't mean *that*. But thanks for reminding me.' Nafisa swigs her orange juice like it's pain-numbing Scotch. 'I mean Dom.'

'Ohhhh.'

Dom has quit psychiatry for a simpler life running a cheese shop. I want to feel happy for him, but I just can't see past the additional gaps it's creating in our out-of-hours rota. Working in the community won't mean I escape doing hospital on-calls.

Nafisa and I are in the bar area of a local comedy club. Whatever Joseph's reservations about humour as a defence, for much of this year it's been our preferred go-to for coping with shitty things.*

'It's strange to think we did Keith's self-defence class twelve months ago,' I say wistfully.

'So how many two-handed shoulder throws did you do this year?' Nafisa asks.

'I came close a few times. But mainly with the bed manager Brian.'

---

* Humour is widely acknowledged as the 'best medicine'. Although for chlamydia, penicillin is still medically preferable to a knock-knock joke.

Nafisa rolls her eyes and busies herself stirring her drink with a straw. She still hasn't forgiven him. I sometimes wonder if it might help Nafisa to talk about her patient who died. Instead she's going with the option of pretending it didn't happen and never mentioning it again. I half-expected that psychiatrists might be better at talking through their feelings. But over the road in the general hospital I know there are also respiratory doctors who hover outside the main entrance on cigarette breaks.

'So, um, do you think we've changed much?' I ask tentatively.

'*Honestly?*' she says, looking at my expanding bald patch.

'Piss off Nafs.'

All she's told me is that the coroner acquitted her of any wrongdoing. The mental health trust did too. It was just one of those incredibly sad things. An occupational hazard of the job.

'Well I guess this is new?' Nafisa says with a half-smile, showing off her sparkling engagement ring. Turns out Nafisa's boyfriend really did want to spend the rest of his life with her. We clink our glasses together again.

Apart from having less hair on my head, I sense I'm not quite the same person either. But more incremental change is harder to see. Like those jaundiced patients from my general medicine days who'd be the colour of Bart Simpson but hadn't noticed because they yellowed just a little bit every day.

'Do you know what you want to specialise in yet?'* she asks, changing conversation.

I shake my head.

---

* As psychiatrists get more senior they can sub-specialise in Perinatal Psychiatry, Child & Adolescent Psychiatry, General Adult Psychiatry or Old Age Psychiatry. There are also sub-specialisms on the 'criminally insane' (Forensic Psychiatry), those with learning disabilities (Learning Disability) and substance-misuse problems (Addictions Psychiatry).

'Well it's going to be *so* much better working in the community,' Nafisa says with a deep sigh. 'More time. Patients who are less sick. Our own consultation rooms. Plenty of tea and biscuits. Apparently it's just like being a GP.'

'Aren't GPs really overworked at the moment?'

Nafisa glosses over this. 'Well it can't be worse than the wards can it?'

After an eventful first half of comedy, the lights go up for the interval and punters spill back out to empty their bladders and refill their glasses. Nafisa hunts for a free table while I queue at the bar. An attractive woman who'd heckled one misogynistic comedian in the first half is standing near me. She has black hair with faded blue tips, big gold hoop earrings and almond-brown eyes with flicks of eye pencil coming from her lids like Cleopatra. Her orange jumpsuit sings against my drab black jeans and charcoal top. If only it were summer, I might have thrown on something more fun like a light grey T-shirt.

'You alright?' I ask. She seems quite drunk, swaying on the spot.

'God, I'm pissed,' she says.

'Can I get you a drink? Maybe a water. Or some sort of IV drip?'

'I'd love some crisps please,' she says. The barmaid hands me some sweet chilli Tyrrell's which I pass on to the woman, who puts them straight into her handbag.

'I'm Benji by the way,' I say, intrigued by this person who seems to think I was offering to restock her cupboard.

'That's a nice name for a puppy.'

'You heckle full-time then?' I say, slightly wounded.

'Sorry, no, I'm an Explainer at the Science Museum. And I'm Esther.'

'That's a nice name for a Second World War widow,' I return volley.

She laughs. 'Singaporeans all have old granny names. Right, I'd better go. Me and my friends might skip the second half so I don't make a dick of myself again.' She scrawls on a beer mat and hands it to me. 'Here's my number if you ever want to take me out for another packet of crisps or something.'

Is that a sign? It's marginally more concrete than wearing yellow or stroking your hair.

I return to our table with my pint and Nafisa's lime and soda. 'What's that?' Nafisa asks when I sit down. I'm still holding the beer mat.

'That, is er, a woman I met at the bar's phone number.'

'Stop mucking about. What is it really?'

Before starting a new job, each year trainees must meet with a so-called educational supervisor to review their progress.

'You almost look too young to be a doctor,' Dr Patel jokes in the staff kitchen while making two enormous cups of coffee, and I'm glad she's too short to see my bald patch. 'Either the trainees are getting younger or I'm getting older. And please, none of this Dr Patel business. Call me Sita.'

We go through to her office where there's an abstract Matisse print on the wall and a spider plant in the corner. We sit down and she gathers a wad of papers and knocks their ends on the desk to align them, with me wondering how we'll get through them all in my thirty-minute slot.

'So Benjamin how has your first year as a psychiatrist been?'

This is the annual dance that doctors have to do, going through the motions, jumping through the right hoops, to get signed off to progress to the next stage of training.

How *has* my first year been? Well, I'm doubting everything and live in constant fear of making a fatal mistake.

'Good thanks!' I say.

There's an unwritten rule in these reviews that the junior doctor will say that they're managing, even if they're not, and the assessor will play along, despite having been through it all themselves and knowing full well how shit it is.

'Pleased to hear it. And has the workload been manageable?' she asks.

It's 7.30 a.m. and we've had to squeeze this meeting in before my twelve-hour on-call shift starts, so I'm pretty sure she knows the honest answer.

She hovers her pen over the 'yes' box anyway, knowing what I'm going to say. Below the 'no' option is just one dotted line for comments, presumably to limit any complaints that are made.

I think of all the evenings working late. The admin done at home in the evenings or at the weekend. The on-calls. And the extra on-calls we inherit when people start leaving. It's a given that you just have to fudge your timesheet and say that you never worked late to comply with the European Working Time Directive (EWTD) of a maximum seventy-two hours so that your employer doesn't look bad.

When I worked in surgery one lad made a fuss, told it like it was, a noble whistleblower speaking truth to power. They failed him.

'The workload has been fine, yes,' I say, along with a completely unintentional yawn.

'Great. Great,' she says, ticking the 'yes' box. 'And how has it been working with Dr Glick?'

I think of Paige, bouncing around in the system, on the wrong floor to be taken seriously. Of the shock therapies we administered which I worry could later join the list of 'barbaric treatments' in the history books. Of the dubious chemical fixes we dish out and the patients we discharged too soon. Of the rapid and thoughtless way we medicalise people without the curiosity or time to dig any deeper.

'Working with Dr Glick has been fine thanks,' I say diplomatically.

Sita smiles and ticks her boxes. 'And are you in therapy?'

I try to do the slow nod of a man who has been in psycho-analysis for some time.

'Oh good,' she says making another mark on the page. 'When did that start?'

'Oh um, just a few weeks ago actually.'

'I'm a big fan of therapy,' she says, coming to life and nodding to a figurine on her desk of Sigmund Freud holding a cigar. 'Can I ask what you're working on in therapy?' She asks the question so casually you'd think Joseph and I were trying to build a model plane together, rather than delve into the deepest corners of my psyche.

'Um, we're trying to work out why I've always wanted to be a psychiatrist.'

'Interesting. Let me know how you get on.' She puts her pen down and leans back in her chair, seeming genuinely interested, and I relax slightly. Maybe this isn't entirely about ticking boxes for Sita. 'And how are you feeling about next year?' she asks.

'Well, to be honest I'm looking forward to working in a less intense environment. The ward could be quite full-on.'

'Community work comes with its own stresses,' Sita says. 'At least in hospital you can lock the doors and windows and keep an eye on your patients. Someone once calculated that even if we see our community patients for thirty minutes every six weeks, that's still something like 99.9% of the time when we're *not* overseeing them. Which leaves a lot of time for things to go wrong.' I try not to think about Nafisa's patient who drowned.

Sita takes a sip from her mug, on which is written: 'You Don't Have to be Mad to Work Here, We'll Teach You'. 'But you'll be fine. The patients will like you. You're calming and you have a nice gentle manner.'

I find it funny when I'm described as 'gentle'. People often say I'm 'calming' too, as if it's something I was born with rather than something I've been forced to learn from somewhere. Also, I'm not sure how to feel as a grown man always being described as 'gentle and calming'. Adjectives you'd usually see on a box of chamomile teabags.

'God, is that the time? Right we'd better rattle through these.' With her thumb, Sita fans the huge wedge of paperwork we still need to complete to 'sign me off'. 'I swear they add more pages every year . . . OK, have you been involved in any SUIs?'

'No, not yet,' I say. SUI stands for serious untoward incidents, which is the medical euphemism for when things go very, very wrong. 'Not since medical school anyway,' I clarify.

Sita leans forward. 'Medical school?'

'I sort of saw one when I was a student but—'

'You saw one?'

'Well, an attempted suicide. I did a placement with the police.'

Sita sits back in silence, hugging her coffee, waiting.

'Well, I remember the message coming in on the radio: man hit by train . . .' I begin.

I can still see it now: Karen the police officer I was shadowing, flicking the blue lights on, hurtling towards the co-ordinates and getting as close as we could which was still miles away. Us climbing the wire fence, litter in the bracken, following the tracks on stone chippings. Running and running towards the bridge in the distance til my calves burned with lactic acid. Me getting there first, Karen nowhere to be seen as she was twice my age and weighed down by all her stuff.

A man in his forties lying across the track, like a sunbather. How it was so weird that he didn't seem in pain, shock maybe. That way he looked up at me.

There were splinters of bone everywhere, he had this hole in the top of his head where the train must have caught him. Blood and something white beneath, either skull or brain. The most surreal thing was that his feet and hands were no longer attached to his body.

'Fuck,' I remember saying.

He kept opening and closing his eyes as he drifted in and out of consciousness. Must keep him talking, I thought.

'You alright mate?' I asked him ridiculously.

He murmured something incoherent, like when someone's sleep-talking.

I am aware that the room is now silent, Sita just watching me.

'I asked him how he got there and he mumbled that he'd jumped off the bridge above us, and when he survived that he crawled on to the railway line. Then he said he'd been run over by a train but still hadn't died.'

I'd looked up at the bridge which must've been maybe fifty feet, as high as the top diving board into a swimming pool with no water in it. I could barely believe he survived the fall, let alone being run over by a train. There was no blood, which someone later told me was because the heat and friction of the wheels cauterises the wounds.

There was still no sign of Karen, so it was just him and me. He said his name was Leon. I took off my jumper and pressed it against the wound on his head. Then I sat down on the tracks and rested my free hand on his shoulder.

I could see the train had stopped a few hundred yards away on the other side of the bridge. The driver was maybe now doing one of those chirpy apology announcements, the passengers huffing and puffing and tutting to one another.

'I asked Leon why he jumped. And he told me that the powers which controlled his body had now set him a "final mission" to save the world by sacrificing himself.'

Sita shakes her head.

'And then Karen eventually arrived and she requested an air ambulance. And the helicopter landed. I'd never seen ambulance crew run over before. They threw my blood-soaked hoody into the gravel, and replaced it with a white sterile pad and bandage. Then Leon was scooped up on to a stretcher and someone gathered up his hands and his feet and put them in a bag.'

You're going to be OK, I told him, having not yet learnt the danger of empty medical promises. And almost as quickly as it had arrived, the helicopter was gone.

Karen and I looked at each other like war veterans who'd seen too much. She apologised for taking so long. I think she even gave me a hug. Someone else asked me how I knew that the train tracks weren't live and I tried to look like it wasn't the first time I'd considered it.

'I got a police bravery award for that at some black-tie event for "actions at the scene of someone who had suffered horrific injuries as a consequence of being hit by a train". Which must be the longest and most specific award title ever created.'

Still Sita doesn't say anything.

It lies somewhere under my bed now because it's not the sort of thing Sam wants hanging in our bathroom.

'The paramedics kept him alive. And the surgeons managed to reattach his hands and feet. But all I could think afterwards was:

what use was any of that if we didn't understand what was making people jump in the first place? It just confirmed to me that I wanted to work in psychiatry.'

Sita nods, gives me her best sympathy face, and hands me a tissue.

What I don't tell her, is that what's threatening to make me cry, isn't reliving this memory, but the sense that the last year has left me further away from understanding the human mind than ever.

PART II

ILLNESS

noun: a disease or period of sickness affecting
the body or mind

12

DR COTTON

'Benjamin let me introduce you to the most important person here,' Dr Cotton says on my first morning at the Wellbeing Centre. He rests an elbow on the front desk. 'This is our receptionist Cheryl. She'll send off all your letters. And she's the only demigod who knows how to operate the photocopier and the fax machine.'

The woman on the phone behind reception beams. She has curly red hair, her hands crossed over her large motherly bosom.

I already like Dr Cotton. He's charming, personable and he doesn't even shorten my name to Ben.

'Benjamin I've asked Cheryl to book up your diary, so you don't have to.'

And he's so helpful too!

Cheryl nuzzles the handset into her shoulder. 'Nice to meet you Benjamin,' she whispers as she hands a leather diary up to me.

Dr Cotton winks from one of his big green eyes, she blushes and returns to her call.

I follow Dr Cotton, his jacket slung over one shoulder, to my clinic room where I'll be based for most of the next year.

'So this is your very own consultation room!' Dr Cotton says.

'Cool!' I say, hypnotised by his enthusiasm and discounting that it's basically a cupboard with a knackered old PC and abandoned coffee cups on the desk growing new strains of antibiotic. It's not too much of a step up from Sam's bedroom under the stairs.

'Feel free to personalise it with plants, family photos, that kind of thing. Have you got little ones?'

I shake my head.

'Married?'

'No. I've got a cactus though.'

'Good for you,' he says.

I idly flick open my new paper diary like a schoolkid on their first day who's just received a fresh workbook. I'm surprised to see patient name after patient name, back-to-back, filling every single white space for months. The first one will be here in half an hour. My chest instantly feels tighter.

'Problem?' Dr Cotton says, looking at me straight-faced.

'Um, I just thought I'd be meeting the team? Maybe shadowing you first?'

'Hit the ground running is what I say! I've got boring management meetings all day and you don't want to shadow me for those, *trust* me.'

'But don't you need to observe me with patients? Just to check you're happy with what I'm doing, and, you know, not dangerous?'

Dr Cotton pats me chummily on the arm 'I'm sure you'll be fine Benjamin, you're in second year now right?'

'Yes but this is my first time seeing patients in the community. You know, alone.'

I'm worried about saying the wrong thing and making the patients *worse* but Dr Cotton presumes I'm talking about safety.

'Just remember, when seeing a patient on your own, always sit closest to the door. Then you have an escape route.'

I scour the architecture of my room. The doctor's desk and chair are by the back wall, and another chair, presumably for the patient, is closest to the door. There's not even a window to climb out of.

'Or,' Dr Cotton continues, 'if that's not possible you can simply press this panic alarm' – he waltzes over to the other side of the room and points at a red button hidden underneath the desk – 'and help will come immediately.'

'*Really?*'

There must be some doubt in my voice and Dr Cotton seeks to reassure me.

'Of course! Let's imagine the worst-case scenario. A patient is blocking your exit, overpowers you and starts to strangle you.' I sense that Dr Cotton has recently done Keith's self-defence refresher course. 'Well if the airway is compromised,' he continues, 'the human brain can survive for what, two to three minutes without oxygen?'

'Uh huh.'

'So once the alarm has been activated, the response needs to be quick. You seem sceptical. Look, I'll show you.' He beeps his watch until it registers the stopwatch function. 'Ready?' he says, grinning. Dr Cotton hits the red button then immediately activates the timer. As the deafening siren rings all around us, his hand hovers expectantly over his wristwatch. We both turn to face the door, and wait . . .

What is going to happen? Are nurses going to burst in with syringes to sedate my hypothetical attacker? Is Cheryl going to charge in and tie them up with a telephone cord?

Eight, nine, ten seconds go by . . . but it probably takes at least that to throw on any body armour or whatever it is our backup is preparing. It's only at thirty seconds, when there is *still* no action at the door, that Dr Cotton's smile starts to fade.

As we hit the one-minute mark, I'm imagining my face turning plum purple as the alarm screeches from the box above us on the ceiling. Dr Cotton starts shifting weight on his feet uneasily.

By two minutes, I'm imagining myself drifting in and out of consciousness, childhood memories flashing before my eyes.

Into the third minute, presumably with me now in a permanent vegetative state, Dr Cotton has seen enough. He storms over to the door, flings it open and looks out into the corridor. I join him to find staff members poking their heads out of their clinic rooms with their fingers in their ears, looking confused.

Cheryl, with her unmistakable red hair, has abandoned reception and is pacing down the corridor towards the exit.

'Cheryl what are you *doing*?' Dr Cotton barks.

'I'm going to file these next door,' she yells with some folders under her arm. 'I can't concentrate with this racket. Is it a test do you think?'

'Yes it's a test!'

'Oh good,' she says, turning around and continuing off in the opposite direction.

We find the maintenance guy who resets the system and the noise stops. He advises Dr Cotton against future unscheduled testing of the system, and says that staff are much more likely to respond to emergency alarms that they're forewarned of.

Dr Cotton marches back to my office, seemingly determined to reassure me. 'Don't worry about that. OK let's imagine, worst-case scenario,' he says again. 'A patient has blocked your path, they're bigger than you and they have a weapon. You hit the panic alarm but no help arrives. What do you do?'

I shrug my shoulders.

'You can offer to get them a glass of water' he says raising his eyebrows and seeming very pleased with himself. 'Then you can exit the room and call for police backup.'

I'm relieved that there's always a contingency plan until I spot a slight hole in the plan. What if the patient doesn't happen to be thirsty? I say as much to Dr Cotton, who scratches his head. 'Um, I think cross that bridge when we come to it. Right, better dash, I'm going to be late for my first meeting. Any problems just give me a call,' he says, rushing off.

As I look around my inevitable death chamber I realise that Dr Cotton hasn't actually given me his phone number.

I tidy up a bit, log into the bulky computer and look at my patient list for the day. Last year I simply had to transcribe Dr Glick's consultations into the notes. Now the potentially life-and-death decisions are on me.

My first patient is attached to a Rottweiler via a metal chain. 'You don't mind dogs, do you?' asks Tariq.

Hands sweaty, heart racing, sweat pricking my back, I feel like I need to escape from the room. Classic fight-or-flight response. 'No no no, not at all,' I gabble. I'm trying to simultaneously give off a vibe of professionalism and to hide the fact that I'm shitting myself and that my desk drawers are full of mouldy coffee cups.

I do have cynophobia, a fear of dogs, but Tariq's referral form says he's seriously considering ending his life, so I want to be as accommodating as possible.

'And he's OK having his treats in here?'

A poster over Tariq's shoulder says 'Strictly no eating or drinking in the consulting rooms' and the canine is already busy working salivary dog-biscuit goo into the carpet.

'I'm sure it's fine,' I say.

There'll be a ten-page hospital-trust dog policy somewhere, but I rationalise it's Tariq's emotional-support pet.

'You sure you're OK with dogs?' Tariq says again. I haven't yet taken my eyes off his furry friend.

For some reason, I decide to come clean. 'To be honest I do have a dog phobia. One attacked me when I was little.'

Aged three, while on a caravanning holiday, I waddled into a guard dog's kennel. A German shepherd chased me out and with its first mouthful it tore the back of my T-shirt like a barber's cape. With its second bite it went to maul me, but at that point was at the full extension of its shackle. My onlooking parents said it was a miracle.

'I can tie him outside if you want?' Tariq offers.

'No it's OK. It's good exposure therapy for me,' I say.

The creature stares at me, no doubt smelling my fear as they always do. His coarse fur coat sits above a robust and muscular body. His teeth are set in liquorice-black gums and crunching through hard snacks like chewing gum.

'Honestly he wouldn't hurt a fly,' Tariq says.

'Probably couldn't hold the newspaper,' I say.

'Eh?'

'Nothing. A bad joke. What's his name?' I ask, clawing at any conversation to distract myself.

'Tyson.'

'After the boxer who bit that bloke's ear off?'

Even Tariq manages a flicker of a smile. 'I can put his muzzle on if you want.'

Why has he got a muzzle?

I tell him it's alright and sure enough my heart is slowing. The principle of flooding or exposure therapy is that adrenaline and anxiety can't stay elevated forever. 'Anyway this isn't really *my* session,' I say, 'I'm supposed to be helping you.'

I begin by checking Tariq's address on our system, which is easy as he doesn't have one. His clothes are soiled, his beard and hair voluminous and matted. All his worldly possessions fit into his rucksack, a cardboard-box mattress bound to it with elastic straps and a sleeping bag bobbing off the bottom.

Tariq might be better suited with the homeless team, but he's attended my clinic today which I see from his file is unusual. I'd risk losing him entirely if I redirected him elsewhere now.

'And your date of birth on our system is . . . oh . . . 31 October 1984. I was born the day before you.'

What next, am I going to divulge my football team, my favourite Spice Girl or some of my juicier family secrets?

I was sometimes critical of Dr Glick's bedside manner, but now I'm learning it's not as easy as it looks. It seems that my consultation style is that of intense oversharing.

'I'm a Halloween baby, yeah. Did your mum leave you in the hospital too?' he says. 'Worst trick or treat ever.'

My mum frequently says the day I was born was the happiest day of her life, just not in front of my three little brothers. I think it's partly because she struggled to conceive me as at the time she was eating only grapefruits and Polos. Anorexia nervosa, F50.0?

In contrast, Tariq was told by a foster parent that after giving birth to him, his alcohol-dependent mother bolted to the pub and never returned. From that first abandonment onwards, his life had been a cruel series of rejections. Kicked out of care homes, schools, low-skilled jobs and council houses, and rejected by society in general, he ultimately swapped domesticity for the reliable chaos of the streets.

'You can't get knocked if you're already in the gutter, can you boy?' he says, patting Tyson's head. 'Dogs don't let you down like humans do.'

Thank God I didn't kick Tyson out.

As he bends forward to ruffle his pet's belly, I get a whiff of alcohol and Tariq confesses that his other best friend is whisky with its dependable numbing effect. 'Like mother like son eh?' he says. 'She was a big drinker, before it killed her. The booze is my connection to her.' He pulls out a mysterious auburn liquid, decanted into a plastic Coca-Cola bottle, today's brown paper bag. 'Do you mind if I . . . ?'

The dog is one thing but I should probably draw a line at people bevving in my consultation room. 'Better not Tariq. Would you tell me a bit about your alcohol consumption?'

Urgh, 'consumption'? So sterile and medical.

'Well some days I spend drinking, other days drinking more. Once I've begged enough for my whisky and Tyson's dog food, I spend the day reading. The libraries usually have central heating.'

'Are there any downsides to your drinking?' I enquire.

He's no doubt had health professionals broach this before.

'Red wine actually reduces your risk of heart disease, you know?' he says.

A slightly lowered risk of heart disease isn't much good with an increased risk of liver disease, gastrointestinal problems, cancer, erectile dysfunction, head injuries and psychiatric disorders. And Tariq doesn't actually drink red wine. He's a three-litres-of-whisky man.

'I'm not that bad,' he says, denial an addict's go-to. Despite his protestations I can see it in his eyes: their giveaway mild yellowing.

'A guy I used to know drank five litres of vodka a day,' he continues.

'What happened to him?'

'I dunno, I've not seen him for a while.'

By reasoning that he's not the biggest alcoholic in the world, Tariq can delay confronting change. I've seen these mental somersaults before. In patients on Daffodil Ward and closer to home. But that *would* be an overshare.

Tariq's also forgetting, or repressing maybe, that his referral stemmed from a walk-in centre he'd attended with stomach cramps where blood tests confirmed early liver disease. Doctors said he was drinking himself to death. Tariq said he sometimes

considered suicide anyway. This prompted the psychiatry referral and I'm still surprised that he came.

'Tariq do you ever feel like life's not worth living?'

'There's nothing for me here. Sometimes I think at least by
dying I might get to meet my mum.'

'Well, no rush, eh? I'm sure she'd be happy to wait for you.'

'That's true,' he concedes.

Protective factors, as Dr Glick taught me, are factors which
prevent a suicidal patient from acting on their death-impulses:
friends, family or partners, strong religious beliefs, a lack of
access to lethal means or an expressed 'cowardice' about following through. The presence of such factors will really help me to
sleep at night.

'Tariq is there *anything* worth staying around for?'

He considers the question. 'Tyson I suppose, I need to be
around to feed him.'

I feel an unfamiliar pang of gratitude for the dog now chewing
my computer's cables.

Time's up.

'Tariq would you consider seeing the specialists at the Drug
and Alcohol Service? Or maybe AA?'

'They don't help,' he snaps.

'I could try and get you an inpatient detox?'

'What's the point?'

An email pings through from Cheryl that my next two patients
are here and becoming agitated.

I just need more time to get Tariq to trust me.

'We have to finish for today but I'd like to refer you to our
team's psychologist. Also maybe next time we could think about
how to inject something else into your life . . .'

*Inject. God, did I just say 'inject'? You've mastered alcohol, now
let's get you on something harder.*

'. . . I'm meaning purpose, by the way. Not, you know. Maybe study or work or something like that. Would you come and see me again?'

Tariq shuffles in his seat about to make an excuse.

'If only to help me overcome my dog phobia?' I add half-joking.

'Yeah, maybe,' he says.

The rest of the day is back-to-back. At 7 p.m. as I'm writing up my GP letters, Cheryl peers into my room, her handbag slung over her shoulder, chewing gum.

'Benjamin I've got to set the alarm now, so maybe finish off at home unless you want to sleep here?'

'Sorry I'm late, flat tyre,' I say, lying down on the couch.

'But why are you *really* late Benji?' Joseph says.

I'm learning that one of the problems with psychoanalysis, with finding meaning in everything, is that the universe conspiring to jam a shard of glass from the road into your bicycle wheel is seen as unconscious resistance to the therapeutic progress.

'I just told you, I got a puncture.'

This isn't the first time we've looked for things that aren't there. Shortly after beginning therapy I developed an itch all over which Joseph rationalised was me struggling to feel comfortable in my new 'skin' as a patient. I later discovered that Sam had just bought us a new biological washing detergent.

'Joseph what's that Freud quote, sometimes a cigar is just a cigar?'

'He never actually said that, it's apocryphal. But maybe you're right. There's a good joke about that actually.' Joseph likes to tell me jokes and fables. 'So a new patient sits down and the therapist waits in silence for ten minutes for them to say something. Eventually he volunteers that his jaw hurts. The therapist quietly ponders; is this a secret too painful even to speak? After another ten minutes of silence the therapist's secretary telephones through: "Sorry to disturb you, that gentleman's meant to be upstairs with the dentist." '

We both laugh together. I'm already fond of Joseph and I'm trying to trust the psychoanalytic process. There's got to be something to it, or else what's in all those books?

A few sessions in, I've now thrown myself metaphorically in the deep end, figuratively on to his couch. I've noticed there's usually a spider that lives on his ceiling and its easier if I pretend I'm just telling it my life story.

Joseph has also been trying to ease my sense of navel-gazing overindulgence. And my nagging guilt that people in the world with serious problems are surely more deserving of my Monday evening slot. Presuming they could afford it. Joseph recently put it to me: 'If someone with a broken leg discovers that someone else has two broken legs, does that invalidate the first person's problems?' So me and my twisted ankle are persevering.

I'm getting better at free-associating, of saying the first thing that comes into my head. In psychoanalysis you don't 'think before you speak', but speak first, and then afterwards make sense of what's been revealed. My first attempts were limited to nouns. I'd say 'Melon . . . wall . . . lamp,' then Joseph would wonder why I'd said melon and I'd explain that I'd had some in my Tesco meal deal. But now I've graduated to free-associating whole sentences while resisting the temptation to rehearse funny or wise tidbits in the waiting room beforehand.

This week, reflecting on Tariq led to me discussing my childhood dog attack. How inevitably everyone remembers it differently. When I broached it with my parents my mum said the T-shirt the dog destroyed was green, which seemed a funny detail to remember. My dad had said that afterwards they'd tried to act normal, as if nothing had happened, so that it wouldn't affect me.

Joseph had said 'interesting' which gave me a dopamine hit and I felt like I was properly 'doing' therapy. This prompted me to tell the story of when my dad worked as a biology teacher at a school seventy miles away and lived down there in our caravan during the week. And how one day my mum telephoned the school to speak to him and the secretary said, 'John hasn't worked here for three months.' He'd still carried on as normal, coming home each weekend as if nothing had happened.

I also told Joseph the story of my mum and her broken wrist which prompted him to say 'It sounds as though your parents like to give the impression of everything being very together, even if their bones aren't,' and I almost wanted to clap.

We talked about how this pretending everything was O K meant that now I sometimes wonder if I've imagined things from my childhood or that I'm going mad. Growing up, whenever I said I was unhappy my mum would say, 'Well it's nothing to do with anything we did, you had an idyllic childhood.'

But there are memories, of banging doors and screaming rows. Of that, and that, and oh God yes that.

After leaving Joseph's, I push my bike along the high street past a photography shop with Kodak moments on display in the window. A family having a pillow fight on a white, fluffy-cloud bed. A child blowing out birthday-cake candles without spit going everywhere. A happy bride walking through a cornfield wearing a wedding dress and stilettos, as you do. Even the picture frames seem like fake wood made with chipboard and a thin oak veneer. I think of my family's photos. Endless happy shots of us building sandcastles. But then my mum did always make us 'smile' before capturing the shot.

I've got a missed call from my mum, no doubt wanting to hear how my new placement is. I don't phone her back.

13

DAISY

I ring the buzzer to Daisy's seventeenth-floor high-rise flat one
final time and am about to give up when I see her coming around
the corner, past the off-licence, the betting shop and some
boarded-up windows, with a Lidl carrier bag in each hand.

'Hi Daisy. Sorry to come unannounced but your phone isn't
ringing so I—'

She puts down a bag and shoots a finger up to her mouth.
'Shhh, it's not safe to talk here.'

In medicine fortunately those with severe illnesses like cancer
are more likely to attend their appointments than those with
something more trivial. As if psychiatry isn't hard enough
already, what with the lack of objective tests or any real cures, in
this speciality I'm noticing that paradoxically it's often the *most*
unwell patients who don't turn up. Why prioritise seeing a stuffy
psychiatrist when aliens are after you?

Daisy was a no-show for her last two appointments with me at
the Wellbeing Centre, a possible red flag that she's deteriorating,
so I've come to her.

She fobs us in and I do as I'm told, staring straight ahead as we
walk to the lift, so as not to arouse suspicion. I feel one briefcase
away from being a secret agent.

Large signs show what is prohibited but courtyard 'ball games'
are probably the least of the estate's problems. A skunky pong
comes from somewhere and inside the lift a notice reminds us:
'Don't urinate in here.'

Any observations I had on Daffodil Ward about the links

between mental illness and poverty have only been confirmed in the community. Lots of my patients live in places like this.

It's often said that 'mental illness doesn't discriminate' and whilst it *can* affect even the princes of England, this seems a slightly misleading sound bite. I'm noticing that it certainly *tends* to disproportionately cling more to low socio-economic status, which seems important to acknowledge when considering prevention strategies. Back on the computer in my box-room office, when creating a new patient profile on our online database, the comprehensive drop-down menu includes titles like Professor, Dame, Duke, Major, Sir, Captain, Baroness, Lady and Right Honourable Lord, but I'm yet to select any of those. Maybe they all just have BUPA.*

Our lift judders to a stop, then as instructed I follow Daisy to her flat in silence.

My mum believes that a person's home reflects their state of mind. 'I don't like chaos, it stops me thinking clearly,' she'd say as she put away the washed-up crockery.

Daisy's letter box is rammed full of serious-looking white envelopes with cellophane windows. She lets us in and puts down her bags. Then she secures all three locks and a door chain. 'OK, it's safe to talk now,' she says.

'Maybe you should open some of those letters?' I say.

'They'll just be from debt collectors and eviction warnings from the council,' she says matter-of-factly.

That's odd, I think.

To the side of the door I notice Daisy's food-splattered white chef Crocs. 'How's work at the cafe?'

---

* Two theories seek to explain this: the causation theory (low socio-economic status breeds mental illness) and the social-drift theory (mental illness leads to a decline in social status).

'Oh, I've quit. I don't have time with all this going on.'

It's dark in the hallway but for a stream of natural light coming from a window ahead of us. I flick the light switch but nothing happens. Maybe it's because of the unpaid bills, or maybe it's because the bulb is encased in enough tinfoil to cook a Christmas turkey.

I follow her to the kitchen which looks like a 1970s sci-fi film set with industrial quantities of tinfoil meticulously covering the light bulbs, the power sockets, the extraction fan and the oven. The electrical kitchen goods including the fridge and toaster have received the same treatment.

'It's to stop him getting my frequency but I've got the other rooms to do,' Daisy explains as she unpacks her shopping bags, another thirty-two rolls of the stuff. 'I'd offer you a cup of tea, but . . .' she says, gesturing to the kettle which is wrapped in three layers of aluminium foil.

On Daffodil Ward I remember another patient's delusions related to metal so maybe there is something to the 'tinfoil' hat stereotype. I wonder now what proportion of profits for aluminium-foil manufacturers is due to psychosis? I just hope psychiatric patients are never directly targeted in their advertising strategy ('Bacofoil – they're watching you!').

Daisy tells me she realised her upstairs neighbour had bugged all of her electrical devices when she returned from a long shift and her toaster had moved a few centimetres further to the right, betrayed by a trail of crumbs. She's switched everything off but it's still happening so now she's wondering if the bugs are embedded deep within the electrical circuit of the entire council block.

I try to keep a poker face and stay calm. 'Daisy I've been trying to call you?'

'I had to destroy my phone,' she says, continuing to empty roll after roll on to the already cluttered table. Among other things on there I notice there's a claw hammer and the remnants of a Samsung.

'Quick, give me yours,' she says, extending her hand to me. 'He could be tracking you.'

Something about handing over my brand-new, uninsured phone doesn't feel like a good idea. 'Um, Daisy do you mind if I just put it on airplane mode?'

I don't want to tell her that I've been texting a woman I met at a comedy club and am awaiting a reply. Well, it's really Nafisa who's been texting Esther for me. We've started revising for our exams in the library together after work. When she learnt that I hadn't texted the beer-mat woman, she commandeered my phone to meticulously compose a message for me. Before deliberately adding some typos apparently so that I wouldn't 'seem like a weirdo'.

This morning I freestyled a text, the first without Nafisa's input, and could see Esther was 'online', then there were those pulsing dots to indicate that she was typing. Then they stopped and she was offline again. Gone. That'll teach me for not running things past my ghostwriter first.

'Turn your phone off completely then,' Daisy says, a fair compromise and I'm relieved it escapes the hammer treatment.

Amongst the clutter on the table are unopened boxes of Daisy's medication, but I'll raise that later.

'It's the upstairs neighbour who's got a problem with me. Same as the guy above me at my last place.' She says it's annoying, as in her application form to be rehoused she said she was flexible about the size, quality and even location. The only stipulation she put on the form was 'no bugs'. I wonder now if the council thought she meant lice. Her eyes dart to the ceiling. 'Listen!'

I wait a few moments in silence, or as close as you get to it in London. 'I can't hear anything.'

'Of course, you can't. He knows you're here. He's clever like that!' she says, tapping her temple.

'And, um, what would you think about coming into hospital?' Daisy is shaking her head before I've even finished my sentence. Most patients hate going into hospital, my uncle always does too.

I scan the room trying to take everything in.

Some things have escaped Daisy's wrapping up: the table and chairs, a fruit bowl and her chopping boards. Also her chef's knives, which are in a quirky knife block in the shape of a human figure, a blade going through each leg, one through the body and another right through the face. It reminds me of something else I should probably ask.

'Daisy do you ever think about confronting this neighbour?'

'No, are you crazy? With the things he says he's going to do to me?'

I instantly relax and take my eyes off the silver blades. 'Yes probably best to leave him alone.'

Sectioning Daisy is an option but being forcibly admitted to hospital is especially traumatic. Daisy does seem quite unwell but the risks aren't *so* high. So I'll just try and help her in the community.

I need to get going as my afternoon clinic is due to start soon. 'Before I go Daisy, could you get a new phone so we can keep in touch?' She says she'll get a cheap one with a new number he can't monitor her on. That was the easy question. 'Also, how would you feel about restarting your clozapine?'

'No no no,' she says, confirming my suspicions that she's long stopped taking it. 'Those meds turn me into a zombie and I need to be alert in case he tries to break in.'

'Fine,' I say, not forcing the issue. You have to pick your battles in psychiatry and being too coercive could just mean she never opens the door to me again. Much better to continue establishing a good therapeutic relationship and gently raise the idea again later. 'Last thing. Would you like me to have a word with the neighbour? Maybe I could mediate.'

She says this would only provoke him, but she does at least agree to me dropping in next week and consents to me calling the housing officer attached to her block.

Back at the office, I call the council's Neighbours Disputes department to try and formally resolve things with the resident of flat 184 above Daisy. They say that that flat's been empty for the last six months while it awaits works, after the previous tenant died there and left it in a right state.

My phone vibrates. A reply from Esther.

I settle into my new routine of seeing patients, staying late to do admin and living with a constant looming fear that I'm going to astronomically fuck up.

When I next visit Daisy, she ushers me in through her front door. There's excitement in her voice. 'Right, I know you think I'm crazy because he was quiet when you were here, but he was so loud last night. I recorded the whole thing.' She reveals a new mobile phone from her pocket and opens the tape-recording app, smiling triumphantly. She presses 'play' and the sound bar starts moving. The silence is shown as a flat line apart from the occasional wave which has picked up her breathing.

Surely that's psychiatric checkmate and I'm now just one question away from Daisy realising she's unwell.

'How do you explain that Daisy?'

'He must've got in here last night and tampered with the tape! I'm going to have to start barricading the front door!' she says, her eyes flashing around the room. In schizophrenia there's always a perfectly irrational explanation.*

'Will you write a supporting letter to the council so I can get rehoused?' she says, eyeing up the furniture.

'Hold on a second,' I say, sitting down on a chair to calm her and also to prevent her from using it as a blockade. She doesn't join me. 'Daisy moving again isn't a long-term solution. Also, I spoke to the council. They told me the tenant above you is, um, no longer there. The flat's empty. Maybe you'd like to see for yourself?'

Part of me is still naively hoping that I can use evidence to convince Daisy that she needn't be scared. Like the adult in horror films who reassures the child that there aren't any monsters in the cupboard and flings open its doors to reveal nothing but coat hangers.

'He says he's going to *kill* me!' she shouts.

The sitting-down really isn't helping.

'How about if I come up with you?'

'No way!'

I'm not sure if this reflects Daisy's fear for this man, or how useless she thinks I'd be in a scuffle.

I tell Daisy that I'm worried about the effect all of this is having on her mental health and she still refuses to restart her medication or to consider coming into hospital. She shows me out, closes and secures the door. Then I hear the ominous sound of furniture scraping across the floor.

Once inside the lift, instead of returning to the ground floor I find my finger pressing the button to '18', one floor above me.

---

* Contrary to what people think schizophrenia isn't a 'split' mind. The most common symptoms are delusions (false beliefs) and hallucinations (seeing, smelling, tasting or most commonly hearing things that don't exist outside the sufferer's mind).

What if Daisy is right? Her fear feels so *real*. It's not out of the realm of possibility that she has an antisocial neighbour upstairs. And some people do get pursued and stalked. Maybe the council lady was looking at the wrong file and was talking about the 184 in a different block. Or maybe there are squatters.

I walk along the bare concrete corridor of floor 18, lots of plain wooden doors with chrome numbers on the front. 180, 181, 182, 183 . . .

I pause a moment outside 184.

What do I expect to find? Some whistling workmen doing repairs? The ghost of the elderly lady who died there? Or a caricature EDL meat-head with an England flag hanging in his window and some suspicious-looking electrical equipment?

I knock but there's no answer.

Back at the office Cheryl is eating a Müllerlight yoghurt at the reception desk, in conversation with Dr Cotton.

'Ah, Benjamin your two o'clock is here,' she says. 'Also, I've just had the police on the phone wondering which doctor just assessed Daisy as fine.'

'I mean she's not fine, but . . . why?'

'Well, they got called to see her and are now taking her to A&E for an urgent psych assessment. Apparently she was walking around her council block with a kitchen knife—'

'*What*?!'

'Nearly electrocuted herself cutting the wires in the communal fuse box. Said she was doing it for the good of the council block but it sounds like other residents didn't necessarily see it that way.'

Dr Cotton raises an eyebrow. I've barely seen him since I started here yet he miraculously seems to have helicoptered in right in time to overhear my mistake. 'Benjamin I'm not sure how you did things on Daffodil Ward, but here we do in the main try to avoid having patients rampaging around the community with kitchen knives,' he says before striding off.

I'm realising that it's not just those with formal mental health diagnoses who think that they can move house to escape their problems.

'How did you feel when your parents moved to the country?' Joseph asks me during my next session.

'I was about seven and I liked it in Newcastle. At least I had some friends. But where we moved to was very remote. My mum worked really hard at making sure we had other children come over to play. But it was generally just me and my brothers and my mum and dad.'

'Hmmm.'

'And everything is just harder. We were basically living on a building site, or in a caravan. Dust and rubble everywhere, no roof initially, no central heating, that sort of thing.'

A recent study I heard reported on the radio found that time in nature improves people's mental health, but there was no mention of the downsides. What they don't tell you about swapping the stress of the city for living in the middle of nowhere is that it's a harsher way of life. The closest neighbour to us was half a mile away, a man with schizophrenia who rarely left his dilapidated house except to try and hitch a lift to Buckingham Palace to get some money from the Queen. And a few miles beyond him were some farmers. Agricultural workers have some of the highest suicide rates, and true to the statistics one day sadly one of them ingested a lethal dose of rat poison. Statistically rural areas have a higher prevalence of mental health problems along with alcoholism and domestic violence.

'And you're cut off socially, geographically isolated,' I continue, 'with no one for miles to gauge what behaviour is normal. Or to check everything's OK if they hear shouting or screaming.'

'Screaming?'

The spotlights in the ceiling look like UFO flying saucers. I wouldn't mind them beaming me out of this conversation.

14

MALCOLM

'We've got a new referral from forensics,' Dr Cotton says during our weekly team meeting. It's one of the few times I ever really see him, or any of my colleagues besides Cheryl. She's sitting in the corner typing up the minutes on a laptop. The highlight of the eye-scratchingly dull weekly meeting is usually when due to a dictation error, instead of being addressed 'Dear psych team' the referrals are addressed 'Dear psychic team'. If *only* we could foresee the future.

I try to stifle a yawn. I woke up last night in a cold sweat following a disturbing nightmare. In it, I was in Nightingale staff car park gassing myself in a car with a hosepipe connected to the exhaust. Through a haze of fumes, I saw a suited man rushing towards me. He knocked on the window and when I wound it down he said, 'Can you *not* do that here? Go and do it in the cemetery car park.' Joseph is going to have a field day with that one.

'He's a gentleman they're discharging from high-security who will need care co-ordinating,' Dr Cotton continues.

Particularly needy or risky patients are sometimes given a 'care co-ordinator'; a named nurse, social worker or occupational therapist who can be their go-to on the phone or in person in between being seen in clinic for medical reviews.

'He's been with them twenty years,' Dr Cotton says. 'I think his index offence was . . .' He scans the paper referral. 'Oh yeah that's it, he killed his mental health support worker. Who wants to take him?'

This is one of the rare times that there's quiet in the NHS. Even Cheryl stops chewing her gum and looks up.

'Come on. If no one volunteers I'm going to have to allocate,' Dr Cotton says. If he gives sole responsibility to me, I may well cry right here in front of the team. My caseload is already dangerously large.

'You promised me you were going to give some of mine to someone else,' one nurse protests.

Dr Cotton identifies the two newest members of the team, Rose who's a nurse and Darrell who's a social worker, who are still building their caseloads. Rose is a slight, softly spoken woman who has the aura and the dainty fingers of a hobbyist flute player. Darrell is so muscular he could probably bench press a piano.

Dr Cotton looks from Darrell to Rose, then back to Darrell. Cogs turning.

'Thank you, Darrell,' he says eventually, handing him the paper referral. 'I'm sure he's much better now.'

After the team meeting we all disperse to see our first patients of the day. Malcolm is a sixtysomething man with unbrushed white hair that grows like the wild hedges he used to trim as a gardener. He's walked to my clinic wearing a fluorescent high-vis jacket due to concerns he'll accidentally bump into fellow pedestrians, but he's never actually hurt anyone.

'Nice to see you again Malcolm,' I say, closing the door and sitting down. 'How are you?'

'Oh I'm fine yes thank you Doctor.'

'Good. What have you been getting up to?'

'Oh you know. Keeping busy. I do my shopping . . .'

I write 'ADL' on my notepad which stands for 'activities of daily living'. This will later go in the notes as evidence that Malcolm is coping on his own.

'. . . I see people,' he continues.

'Oh great, who do you see?'

'Just you really.'

I've met Malcolm only once before, at his clinic appointment three months ago. He's generally been seen in clinic so infrequently because he's what overworked psychiatrists describe in the notes as 'doing well', although we set a low bar here. As I firefight against new referrals being added to my bulging caseload, I'm often just satisfied if patients with serious mental illness aren't endangering themselves or others.

I know Malcolm went into hospital the first time in his twenties with a fiancée by his side but came out eight months later alone. Initially, relatives visited frequently. But with subsequent admissions, the visits became weekly and then monthly and then dwindled to nothing.

'Malcolm, do you ever feel lonely?'

He considers for a moment. 'If I'm honest, I do yes Doctor.'

'I'm sorry to hear that. How does a typical day look for you then?'

'Well, I ride the buses on my Freedom Pass. I like the number 9 and the 24. They're nice routes to look out of the window. I sometimes chat to people or to my voices. That sometimes scares people though.'

'Why do you think it scares them?'

'I think they worry I'm going to hurt them,' he says looking down at the floor. 'So I usually just go for walks now.'

'Great! Where do you like walking?'

'Just around my house really.'

'Oh. As in, up and down the stairs?'

'No, my route is that I go from the living room to the kitchen. Then from the kitchen to the living room. Then from the living room to the kitchen, and I just sort of keep doing that.'

'Oh,' I say again. 'Maybe try a local park to get some fresh air?'

'That's not a bad idea, thank you very much Doctor.'

Emails ping through from Cheryl, my next patient is here.

Unlike Damien the car-thief 'voice-hearer', Malcolm has been in no hurry to mention his symptoms, and I don't get the sense that he's trying to convince me that he's mentally ill. Also tellingly he says he hears the voices coming from *outside* his head. Classic schizophrenia.

Before finishing I ask my usual safety-netting questions: do the voices tell Malcolm to hurt people? Is he thinking of killing himself? He says no to both, wincing as he does, and I apologise for having to ask them.

'I'll be off then,' he says somewhat abruptly. I'd probably be miffed if psychiatrists assessed my likelihood of suicide and homicide every time they met me too. 'See you again in three months?' he says.

With the system so stretched it's tempting to see such low-risk patients infrequently, every three, six or twelve months or even discharge them back to their GPs. I've reassured myself that Malcolm's life isn't endangered. But there's a difference between being alive and living.

I imagine Malcolm rambling around his house alone for the next ninety days. Potentially not hearing another human voice other than the burbling of the radio or small talk with a supermarket cashier. And even then he might get a scan-and-pack machine.

'Let's make it three weeks shall we Malcolm?' I say, squeezing an appointment into a lunch break. He writes the date down in his small paper diary as I know he doesn't have a phone. 'In the meantime, I wonder if you'd like to get involved with some outdoor groups or volunteering. I know you've got green fingers from your previous job and there's a community garden not far from you.'*

'Oh yes, that does sound good,' Malcolm says in his likeable, almost childlike way.

'Excellent. Well, since you're here I'll refer you now so they know to expect you.' I call the number with Malcolm patiently waiting.

'Hello Juniper Community Gardens!' says a sunny voice on the other end of the line, an advert for the restorative power of gardening.

'Hi I'm Benjamin, a doctor in the area. I'd like to refer a patient who's keen to volunteer with you please.' Malcolm and I smile at each other.

'Fabulous!' she says and I imagine her surrounded by sunflowers. 'We currently have several patients helping and we always welcome extra hands! Which hospital are you calling from?'

'The Wellbeing Centre which is a community hub affiliated with the Nightingale Hospital.'

'Oh,' she says. It isn't the 'oh' that ends on a high intonation when you discover you've actually got an extra day of annual leave, but its lower-pitched cousin, like when you discover you're on-call over Christmas.

'Do we not come under your area?' I ask. Malcolm's face falls slightly.

---

* The therapeutic benefits of horticulture have seeded a new treatment called eco-therapy. 'Social prescribing' is now in vogue, and a Manchester GP practice achieved just as good results for depressed patients with communal gardening as with Prozac. Ever the disciple of biological psychiatry, Dr Glick said 'The microorganisms in the soil must have an antidepressant effect on brain chemistry.' My hunch is that the healing comes from being in nature, having purpose and connecting with others, more than any magical microbial mud.

'Um yes you do but um . . . isn't that the *psychiatric* hospital?'

'Yes.'

'So they have a psychiatric diagnosis?'

I cough a few times, conscious of Malcolm's presence, grateful that he's hard of hearing.

'He has schizophrenia, yes,' I say, but not quietly enough and Malcolm flinches. 'But that's definitely not the most interesting thing about him,' I add, giving Malcolm my cheeriest smile. 'Also, he was a professional gardener before he became unwell so it would be mutually beneficial.'

'*Schizophrenic*,' the woman says, chewing the word over in her mouth like a toffee, threatening to extract a filling. The same word my own grandfather struggled to accept for his son, my uncle Thomas. 'It's just, Doctor, you do know, we are an open garden?'

'I do.'

'So, and I'm sorry to have to ask, would he be safe around members of the public?'*

I'm just glad I didn't put this call on loudspeaker. Malcolm is such a gentle soul that the only life forms that need worry about his garden visit are the weeds. I take a deep breath. 'He would, yes. And you're a community garden and he's a member of your community.'

---

* Most violence is committed by people *without* mental illness. But to many, the word 'schizophrenia' has bloody and disturbing associations. This risk is exaggerated by unhelpful, sensationalist tabloid headlines which plaster words like 'schizo', 'psycho' or 'nutter' on their front pages on the rare occasions that someone with the diagnosis is violent. In reality people with schizophrenia are more likely to be victims of violence. Alcohol and drug misuse is a far bigger risk factor for violence and homicide, yet curiously people don't fear parties like they do psychiatric hospitals.

She pauses for a moment. 'OK fine. He can drop by on Tuesdays any time between 11 a.m. and 4 p.m.'

'Thank you,' I say, writing down the details.

'Before you go, Doctor, could I get your name and number? Just in case we need to contact you in an emergency.'

After putting down the phone I turn to Malcolm. 'They can't wait to meet you!' I say, but he doesn't look particularly convinced. 'Pop in any time on Tuesdays between 11 a.m. and 4 p.m. and I look forward to hearing how you get on.'

'It's impossible to tell just by looking at someone if they're going to be violent,' I reflect with Joseph. With Malcolm still on my mind, I'm free-talking in my now familiar horizontal position. 'Society expects certain people to be violent, and many of them never will be. And conversely, some people that you would never expect to be are violent behind closed doors.'

Joseph makes himself comfortable in his chair. 'Tell me more about that . . .'

We'd all sit at the kitchen table, me and my brothers still in our school uniforms, our mum in her stylish, professional psychology workwear and our dad still wearing his blue overalls. He'd serve the food he'd made, usually a tasty vegetable casserole.

As we ate, one of us would ask our mum about her day and she'd say, 'Oh, well I will just tell you about it actually, it's quite interesting,' as if it were a novelty to be asked, rather than how many evening meals played out. And so we'd listen to the tale of the latest severely disturbed child, someone born with no eyes or ears, or cerebral palsy, or autism, or a severe brain injury, my mum talking so much she'd forget to eat. I don't think psychologists were meant to discuss their cases but she never used their names.

At some point she would refill her empty wine glass right to the brim. 'Do you think you could get any more in there, Abi?' my dad would try to joke. Then he'd ask her to please eat her food whilst collecting our empty plates and putting them in the sink. He'd take away the bottle of wine too, trying to do so casually.

'Do you mind?' my mum would snap.

'I think you've had enough love,' he'd say.

'I've only had two glasses.'

'Well there was another bottle in the fridge before.'

'I don't know what you're talking about,' she'd say dismissively.

Once when my dad asked where a bottle had vanished to, my mum quite creatively said she'd been 'cooking with it', and that evening we had baked potatoes. Most of the time she'd buy boxes of wine partly because they're cheaper but also I suspect because it kept her consumption ambiguous.

Sensing an attack, my mum would fight back, with evidence of something else that had gone missing – a chocolate brioche, or slice of fruitcake or some other exhibit of my dad's failing diet. Despite doing manual labour all day and only having tiny portions when we ate together, his waistline mysteriously never seemed to shrink. Maybe it was just his constitution, he'd say. Although once when he returned to the table from the fridge he had a brilliant white moustache, which he hastily wiped away from his top lip when I told him. And I don't think you can blame a slow metabolism on drinking double cream directly from the pot.

My mum's diet wasn't always that healthy either. She used to be very thin and lived off lettuce leaves and reduced-fat salad cream. For lunch she would have half an apple.

In private my dad would always tell me that he only comfort-ate because of my mum, and she'd sometimes say that she only drank because of my dad. Blame ricocheting around our house like a hot squash ball.

My brothers and I would try to move things along. But her blood would be up now and she'd ask what my dad had done that day. He'd tell her he'd replaced the rotten bathroom floor, or fixed a leak in the roof, or insulated some walls or whatever it was. And she'd remind him that they were meant to have been done six months ago. She'd be catching up now, putting forkfuls of salad into her mouth.

'If you got some help, then maybe you could have a full-time career like most men. There's more to life than bricks and mortar. This isn't the life I signed up for when I married you,' she'd say. They both always said the same things, word for word. My dad asking my mum not to drink, shout or speak unkindly. My mum asking him to lose weight and get a job. Neither of them seemingly able to.

At some point my mum would turn to us. 'Boys, can you imagine how stressful it is being married to someone who earns no money? Someone who has no job and no income?' My dad would get up, bring over some yoghurts for dessert, and sit back down again. 'And whose sister never speaks to him.'

My dad would quietly absorb all this stuff. Never crying or letting the pain show until it was too late.

My mum would then get up to put her plate in the sink, and return with the bottle of wine.

'I think you've had enough Abi,' my dad would say.

'What's that supposed to mean?'

'Well you're just starting to get a bit angry and raise your voice.'

'I'm not raising my voice!' she'd yell. 'So I can't even have one drink after work? I pay for the food and wine. I pay for everything in this house I don't even want to live in.'

She'd go to pour another glass, the final straw for my dad. He'd lean over the table, and grab her by the wrist with a burly hand. We couldn't always position them quite far enough away.

'Enough!' he'd bellow.

My mum would eyeball him. 'Or what are you going to do, hit me?'

On the good days, he'd release his grip. The crisis temporarily averted.

'OK, I'll be getting on in the barn if anyone needs me,' he'd say, and already wearing his work clothes, he'd go outside.

'Honestly boys, sometimes I really don't know what's wrong with·your father,' my mum would say, filling up her wine glass.

'So *that's* why you left the relationship-history bit blank,' Joseph says.

'Huh?'

'On the new-patient questionnaire. Most men your age who come in here never stop talking about sex.'

'Sorry I'm not juicy enough for you Joseph.'

'It's just an observation.'

Today Joseph is really leaning into the stereotype that psycho-analysts really only care about one thing. And it's odd being told you lack sexual dynamism by someone in a brown cardigan.

I have for whatever reason had a distinct lack of relationships myself. It seems to bemuse people who like to tell me that I'm not even bad-looking.

Maybe it's because growing up I saw that whatever my parents did to each other, they would never break up. So unconsciously I think that it's safer not to get stuck in anything. My parents do seem to love each other unconditionally, but it's admittedly a messy blueprint for love.

'You don't have relationships because you fear you'll be violent,'

Joseph tells me. 'It's not uncommon for those who've grown up around what you have. You're so anxious about repeating the cycle that you're overcompensating. You infantilise yourself as nice little boy Benji who doesn't do adult things like fucking.'

I stop myself asking Joseph if he could just call it a naked cuddle.

It's true that growing up I always vowed I wouldn't repeat the explosive mistakes of my dad. A promise I've kept good on, but admittedly that has come at the cost of avoiding romantic relationships. Well, apart from Nina.

I tell Joseph about my ex-girlfriend from medical school who visited my family home once. It didn't start too well; as Nina was saying hello to my brothers in the hallway my mum whispered in my ear, 'She's not the one for you sweetheart.' Nina hadn't even managed to take her coat off.

We broke up shortly after that, after trying to be grown-ups going for a weekend together in Porto. Nina was beautiful, complicated and always wore black, rocking the funeral-chic look even by the poolside. A sunbathing goth. We'd try reading together and then after ten minutes she'd get in the water. So I'd hop in with her and she'd quickly climb out. When I joined her back on the loungers, she'd go and sunbathe on a deckchair at the other end of the pool. It looked like I was harassing her, so I had to reassure onlookers that we had actually come on holiday together.

'You choose people with avoidant attachment styles like your own so that you won't feel smothered or claustrophobic. Those who will stay at arm's length, or even a swimming pool's length away. As you were talking I was imagining you both as a pair of hedgehogs who crave intimacy but daren't get close.'

Joseph helps me to see how, yes, perhaps growing up trying to stop your parents from seriously hurting each other could potentially impact on your own future relationships. Especially if it's been kept secret.

'Did anyone else know what was going on at home?' Joseph asks.

'I think my grandparents knew. They were always involved in crisis talks about their relationship. But what could they do?'

'Did you ever think about going to the authorities?' Joseph asks.

'A few times. But never seriously,' I say.

'What stopped you?'

'I guess because my dad is essentially a good person. But one who sometimes did bad things. I just think living in the wild can sometimes send people that way.'

I reflect on the loving memories I have from when I was younger; of the lifelike birthday cakes he'd make and the Ladybird bedtime stories he'd read to me where he'd covered the scary witches' faces with masking tape. And when my favourite soft toy lost its stuffing how he'd take it into 'hospital' for an operation, and when I woke up he'd sewn Bear up again. Acts of service are my dad's 'I love you.' He would do anything for us boys and my mum, and even now on the rare occasion we all watch TV together, he'll still always say he prefers to sit on the floor so we can have a sofa-seat. Anything, that is, except abandon the building project that has become his life's work and move back into civilisation.

When we were snowed in and my dad dug me out so I could get to work, ploughing the snow off the hill that leads down to our house and the bridge at the bottom, I wondered 'can I really recall that horrible thing that once happened here?' And when we returned the tractor to the barn afterwards, going past the tree house he built for me and my brothers, I thought 'Can that mad memory I have from here honestly be true?'

Disturbingly, as part of my exam revision I've learnt that violence often passes through the branches of a family tree like knotweed. And I've plotted enough genograms to see history repeating itself and the victims growing into the perpetrators.*

'Well, you come here. And you are not your dad.'

I don't share Joseph's confidence, and not just because I grew up with my mum saying 'God, you're just like your father.' With time I've come to resemble my dad, from the beard to the balding. I've pushed in vain against the latter, almost seeing it as a metaphor for my transformation into him. Dr Waterhouse and Mr Hyde.

'I think if you dared get into a relationship you might surprise yourself. Have you not had *any* love interests in London?'

'Not really.' I think about Esther. 'Although, I have been texting a funny girl I met at a comedy club a few weeks ago. But we haven't met up. I've been too busy trying not to get struck off, you know?'

'I think that's just an excuse Ben.'

'My name isn't Ben,' I say, managing to mask most of my irritation. 'It's Benji or Benjamin. How many months have I been seeing you now?'

The problem with having an old, wise therapist is that he can also be forgetful. Joseph sees patients back-to-back and doesn't ever make notes, so he often forgets the basics, confabulates for gaps in his memory or muddles up details from my life story with his other patients.

---

* In the famous 'Bobo Doll Experiment', children who witnessed violence towards a doll were more likely to mimic it themselves, along the principles of so-called social learning theory. There are also biological risk factors beyond a person's control, so-called monoamine oxidase-A 'warrior genes' hidden in a person's DNA. So if nurture doesn't get you, maybe nature will.

When I last shared my frustration with Nafisa during one of our revision sessions, she told me that her therapist once asked if she ever worried about becoming a heroin addict like her brother Ahmed. Nafisa doesn't have a brother, and certainly none of her family use opiates. But at least her therapist knows her name.

'Sorry *Benji*,' Joseph says now with emphasis, as though depressing the sticky bit of a mental Post-it note which will fall off again later.

'Look Benji, I know work is busy but do you think that stops other doctors having relationships?'

It's true that most of my friends from medical school are now either in long-term relationships or married. Nafisa's engaged. God, the rumour is that even Dom's got a partner now.

'Not surprising that you're avoidant in love, but life is short. Look, I'm not supposed to be too directive in therapy but take it from an ageing man off the record: you're young, you're not that bad-looking . . .'

This again?

'. . . and these are supposed to be the best years of your life. Get out there into the world!'

I'm not sure how I feel about this new alpha-male version of Joseph. But on the bright side, he does also forget to bill me for my session.

15

ESTHER

'Sorry I'm late!' Esther says when she arrives from work at the Science Museum, still wearing the iconic red polo shirt. 'OK Benji you should probably know, I'm late for everything. I optimistically think I can squeeze in another thing and then I lose track of time. But I've only ever missed two flights,' she says proudly. 'They always call your name over the tannoy first you know?'

'Esther remind me to never go on holiday with you.'

'You're not one of those squares who's at the airport two hours before, are you?'

'No,' I say, shaking my head. 'I like to be there the full recommended three hours before.'

With a nudge-cum-shove from Joseph, I'd arranged to meet Esther after work. Following my session, all geed up I'd sent the text. It turns out that sometimes it really is as easy as asking if someone's free on Friday night.

I got here early so ordered us some drinks and snacks and realised I'd chosen a pub in Elephant and Castle that's on one of the UK's largest roundabouts and blares rock music even in the early evening. Someone from the kitchen brings over our chips and some condiments.

'Enjoy your food!' the waitress says.

'You too!' I say, a combination of nerves and deafness, which seems to amuse Esther.

'Should we go somewhere quieter?' I yell. She nods and we find an outside table amongst the road rage, revving engines and air pollution instead.

'I didn't have time for lunch today,' she says, dunking chips in mayonnaise. 'So you're a doctor, that's so impressive!'

'Hah, not really. I went to Leeds Medical School whose most famous alumnus is Harold Shipman.'

'Oh.'

'At least at my medical-school interview I knew if I didn't get in I could always tell myself they're not always the best judge of character.'

It's a stupid joke that I've cracked before but it feels nice to make her laugh.

She continues attacking the French fries. 'So how's your work? It must be so rewarding helping people.'

I can't stop thinking of Malcolm riding the buses alone, or doing laps of his house. But it doesn't really feel like first-date chat. 'Yeah work is fine,' I say, nodding slightly too vigorously.

'Do you enjoy it?' she asks as she chews.

'Enjoy' isn't quite the right word for that constant anxiety that something absolutely horrendous might happen. After seeing the benign soul that was Malcolm I had thought that I might actually sleep easily for once. But even with him I can't stop wondering if the woman on the phone was right and if Malcolm is currently wreaking havoc with some hedge shears. I can see the tabloid headlines: 'BONKERS PENSIONER GOES ON RAMPAGE DECAPITATING FLOWERS IN COM-MUNITY GARDEN.'

I cradle my empty pint glass. 'Do you fancy another?'

'Yeah, go on,' she says, taking a big gulp of wine. 'But I'll be a good feminist and get these ones. Although, you are a rich doctor and I'm skint,' she says with a twinkle. 'I'll come in with you though and see what they've got.'

The crowd at the heaving bar is three rows deep, with a couple of tattooed, stern-looking barmen behind it. Eventually one of them motions to me.

'Esther what do you want?'

She leans forward on the bar, scanning the fridges. 'Have you got any white wines that taste like gooseberries?' she asks the barman. For an almost unbearable five minutes she makes him get out all the bottles of white wine and she peers at the labels. Then she asks if she can try two of them, sipping them thoughtfully. 'Actually I'll just have half a cider please.'

I shake my head, laughing.

'Don't ask, don't get,' Esther says sitting back down. 'And I want to like it if I'm paying £9, sorry if you're paying £9 for a small wine. Besides, he was rude. And shy bairns get nowt. You should know that as a fellow Geordie,' she says.

That's weird, I think. 'Um, how do you know I'm from Newcastle?'

Esther looks into her cider. 'OK this is awkward. I was going to tell you. Oh fuck, how to say this without sounding like a weirdo . . .'

I sit up straight. Why when I meet someone nice does there have to be a catch?

'Basically when we met, I went to that comedy club knowing you'd be there.'

Oh great, a stalker.

'My mum and your nan sort of set us up.'

A surprised laugh escapes from my mouth. 'Esther what are you on about?!'

She tells me that when my grandpa was still alive, he would always go to a philosophy evening class in Newcastle, which is true. Apparently Esther's dad also attended and when they realised they shared a wedding anniversary the two couples sometimes celebrated it together. When my grandpa died, Esther's parents continued the tradition, by going round to my granny's for a meal so she wouldn't be alone just with her carers on her wedding anniversary.

'Now they're friends and my mum was telling your nan that I live in London and only ever meet dickheads. And your nan said you live here and are always, usually single.'

I try not to go the colour of the buses I can see over Esther's shoulder.

'So my mum told me your name and I found you on Facebook. And you looked sweet. And then I saw you'd clicked "attending" to that comedy night, so I dragged some friends along. I was dead nervous, that's why I drank a bottle of wine. Then I gave you my number and it only took you this long to ask me out.'

I just sit there is silence, still half-expecting her to slip up with every next sentence.

'So are you going to get a restraining order against me?' she says to the ashtray.

I sip my beer and wipe the froth from my top lip.

'Say something Benji? Do you think I'm really creepy?'

'I'm just a bit surprised,' I say, dispirited that on the rare occasion that I get a girl's phone number it's only because of my wingman grandma.

'Well you look disappointed,' she says hurt. 'Just remember that you spoke to me first.'

'How did you get on with the gardening Malcolm?' I enquire, back in my clinic, several weeks later.

'Oh I didn't actually go, Doctor. I didn't really feel like it.'

Maybe it's the 'negative symptoms' of his schizophrenia: the characteristic apathy and amotivation which comes later in the illness. Maybe it's his energy-sapping antipsychotic medication quetiapine or the obesity and diabetes that it's given him. Or maybe it's because after a lifetime of seeing the look in people's eyes when he mentions the word 'schizophrenia', he knows he isn't really welcome.

Before Malcolm leaves, I ask if he'd like to increase his quetiapine dose to help quieten the voices. 'No thank you doctor,' he says. 'Some of them are nice. And besides, they keep me company.'

16

PAIGE

On Sunday morning I'm on-call again and the huge whiteboard of psychiatric referrals is already full of names, so the second board is out. Never a good sign.

I now sometimes see simpler cases first as it helps psychologically to cross off some names early doors. I begin with a familiar one, reasoning I can discharge her quickly.

I enter Bay 7 in A&E to find an emergency doctor suturing Paige's self-harm wounds. She's wearing last night's summer dress with the instantly recognisable 'Mam' and 'Dad' tattoos on each arm in their smudged, pale red hearts.

Yesterday she added a new word to her collection, slicing it deep into her thigh with a carving knife, past the epidermis and the dermis and into the subcutaneous fat beneath. With her legs outstretched on the bed, the skin flops out unnaturally on each side, creating gaping white gashes like shark attack injuries I've seen in photos.

Non-lethal self-harm is sometimes dismissively called a 'cry for help', but it can be an attempt to communicate pain. Sometimes the message is easier to understand than others and the poker-faced doctor is a model of professionalism as she traces the angles of Paige's four-letter expletive with her needle and suture. Starting with the 'C'.

'Morning Paige. I'm Benjamin the on-call psychiatrist this weekend. We've met a few times now.'

Paige looks up briefly from playing Candy Crush on her phone. 'Oh, it's you.'

I remember the first time I met Paige with Dr Glick when she was considering jumping from her second-floor flat window. Back then I'd railed against the uncaring system, if only in my head. Vowed that I would do better.

The second time we met was when her boyfriend kicked her door down just before Christmas and I got in Dr Glick's good books for discharging her so decisively.

Since then I can see from the notes that she's seen multiple psychiatrists. The most recent entry is from Nafisa:

```
Patient attended A&E saying she was going
to kill herself this evening but tell-
ingly came with an overnight bag packed.
When I refused admission she pulled a
handful of paracetamols from her pocket
and put them in her mouth. She then asked
for a glass of water and was angry when I
refused. She then tried crunching them
but too dry and she ended up spitting them
out. Finally she tried to throw the
weighted A&E furniture at me, but unsuc-
cessful. She stormed out stating that
she'd made her point.
```

And now, Paige is back. In an ideal world I'd wait for the doctor to finish patching her up, but several other patients in A&E are already dangerously close to breaching the holy 'four-hour target'.

'Paige can I ask you some questions about last night?' I say. 'It might take your mind off the procedure.' The suturing doctor is now sewing up the U.

'I like the pain,' Paige says. People who self-harm sometimes say pain is a welcome 'release' for overwhelming emotions.

'Well could we talk anyway? Maybe if you could stop playing that game?'

She finishes her round of Candy Crush, a celebratory chime signalling a new high score, then lowers her phone. Paige looks at me for the first time with her familiar sea-blue eyes.

'Thank you. So what happened last night then?' There's a slight irritation in my use of the word 'then', a new tone I'm using increasingly frequently, impatient to start discharging – sorry, assessing – all the others.

'I dunno. I just remember the pigs turning up and then being here. I wasn't doing anything! I'm never the one doing anything! Is it normal to have pain here?' she says pointing accusingly to where the barbs hit her chest.

'Yes, I think it's pretty normal to be sore after being tasered.'

She looks at me sceptically. 'Well, it didn't hurt this much *last* time.'

Last night, according to the notes Paige had called 999 distressed and threatening suicide. She gave police the address of her second-floor flat and on their arrival, encouragingly she wasn't consuming heroin. She was chugging vodka though, with bloody legs and a blade to her throat. When she refused to put it down, police disarmed her with a taser.

'The police report says they were worried you might seriously hurt yourself. Do you remember having a knife to your neck?'

'Not really.'

'Does it sound like the sort of thing you might do?' I ask.

'I don't know, do I? But I'm fine now. I'm not gonna kill myself. I just need to get home. My boyfriend's coming round later.'

I'm relieved she's not angling for an admission this time, which makes my life easier and means I'll avoid any more rude emails from ward consultants querying my 'inappropriate' use of a hospital bed by giving it to someone who isn't really, really unwell.

But I still need to check Paige is safe to discharge. Besides it looking good professionally that none of my patients have killed themselves, a strange gold star on my curriculum vitae, God knows how I'd cope emotionally if it ever happened.

'Paige, can I ask what's changed from a few hours ago?'

'I've had some sleep, I've sobered up. And he texted me back.'

Paige has continued her habit of a lifetime by having relationships with abusive men who afford her the quality of love she thinks she deserves.

'That time he kicked your door in you said you were going to leave him,' I say.

'I can't. It's complicated.'

That word again. Isn't it ever.

'Do you remember doing your leg?'

'Yeah I did that earlier in the day when he wasn't replying.'

I can relate to the distress of having no texts or when getting no reply from Esther despite seeing those bloody blue ticks. And my own brain will sometimes even goad me when I'm standing on the side of a busy main road.

No one would miss you, you know?

All that bullshit. But the worst thing I've ever actually done is send five additional texts to Esther checking everything's OK. A feature of Paige's diagnosis – emotionally unstable personality disorder, sometimes known as borderline personality disorder, and likely born of an attachment problem in her early life – is a low tolerance of frustration which means that small stressors can evoke big reactions. Something will unsettle her and she'll cope by turning to drugs, drink or self-harm or consider stopping the pain altogether through suicide. She'll come in intoxicated and distressed, sometimes she'll need treatment for overdoses and other times her only medicine is simply a hot chocolate, a sandwich and a sleep. Then in the morning she'll usually be alright again and feel ready to leave hospital.

I note the patchwork of older, paler, self-harm scars on her forearms. 'Next time you get the urge to cut yourself, could you try something else?'

'Yeah, yeah eating chillis, squeezing ice cubes, pinging elastic bands off my skin and all that other crap you lot suggest. None of it works.'

'I could ask the crisis team to call you later?'

'Now they *would* make me suicidal,' she says.

The suturing doctor sighs audibly, cramp or is it annoyance, then continues with her task.

'Some people find therapy helpful?' I try.

'No no no, I just need to go home.'

I'm mildly relieved that she's refused therapy too since she may not even be eligible. The few precious places for NHS dialectical behavioural therapy (DBT) – the long-term model that can help so-called emotionally unstable personality disorder which takes some ideas from CBT – are reserved for the most chaotic and dysfunctional patients. Even if you're gouging obscenities into your thigh you may not qualify. It's rarely available instantly either.

After Tariq hadn't objected to the idea of talking therapy, I referred him to our psychologist at the Wellbeing Centre and asked where he was on the waiting list. She consulted her Excel spreadsheet. 'Well, he's currently eighty-third so I'd usually get to him in a year or two,' she said. 'But I'm leaving soon and they haven't found a replacement yet so it could be a bit longer.'

'All finished here,' says the doctor, cutting the ends of the dissolvable suture threads from the 'T'. Paige's skin is now sewn back together with chunky white stitches like the side of an American football.

'We can discharge you then,' I announce with a smile. 'Can I call someone to come and take you home?'

'Like who?' Paige says.

I glance at her arm tattoos. 'Maybe your mum? Or your dad?'

'My mam's dead and my dad used to abuse me, so I'm OK.'

'Oh yes, sorry.'

I dimly remember how it felt to hear Paige's tragic story for the first time on Daffodil Ward. But since then I've heard hundreds of others and now the misery has just blended into one.

'Maybe your boyfriend could come and collect you?' I continue, keen to pass responsibility on to someone else.

'He'll be playing Xbox,' Paige snorts.

She winces as she gets off the bed with her fresh stitches. Then she shoves me out of the way, so that I bang against the yellow clinical-waste bin. 'You're not new any more, are you?' is her parting shot.

'Don't mention it madam,' says the emergency doctor once Paige has gone, removing her blue gloves with a snap.

I'm now used to rarely being thanked and I've been shouted and screamed at far more times than I've heard the hallowed two-word phrase.

'How do you lot deal with all these PDs?' the emergency doctor continues, now washing her hands. 'PD' is the commonly used, usually pejorative, shorthand in mental health for 'personality disorder'. Many people won't even give them the time to say their diagnosis in full.

Women are known to be disproportionately diagnosed with borderline personality disorder. A paper once published in the *British Journal of Psychiatry* was even entitled: 'Personality disorder: the patients psychiatrists dislike'. Instead of being celebrated as survivors of abuse, women like Paige are dismissed as having 'disordered' personalities and kicked out as quickly as possible.

'Well, we don't really deal with them do we, it's all a bit hopeless.'

'She gets stamped in here more than my Starbucks loyalty card. She'll be back in a few days when she has a fight with her boyfriend or no one likes her Instagram post. If she really wanted to kill herself, she'd just do it wouldn't she?'

When A&E is forever overwhelmed, some healthcare workers get frustrated by patients who seemingly do-it-to-themselves. And unlike on British Airways, 'frequent flyers' in hospital rarely get upgraded to a better service. I try to remember that patients like Paige have usually had shitty early lives that affect how they cope as adults. And that rejecting them now, merely reinforces that. Also, people with personality disorder do have an increased risk of eventual suicide. And if butchering yourself with a kitchen knife is a *relief* from your emotional pain, how bad must that be?

I dispose of the crumpled blue paper tissue Paige was lying on, then I pull a fresh length down on to the bed for the next patient.

The doctor is still scrubbing her hands as though trying to wash off the uncomfortable feelings projected into us by Paige, which psychoanalysts call 'countertransference'. 'I really don't know how you stay calm with people like that who are so up and down,' she says.

I've had a bit of practice, I think.

I'm talking to Joseph about the comment my disinhibited, matchmaking grandmother made when I first told her I wanted to be a psychiatrist: 'How can you have any faith in that nonsense when your mum is the way she is?'

'Do you think there's anything in that stereotype of the professionals being as mad as their patients?' I ask.

Joseph laughs. 'Sometimes, yes. Do you?'

'Maybe. But strangely with my mum it was always her work that pulled her through.'

Joseph straightens his trousers as you do in the cinema before a film starts. 'Go on . . .'

I recall to Joseph a time when my mum was lying on the floor saying that she wanted to die. Which was a shame because for ages she'd been saying that all she needed to be happy was a VW Beetle. And a fortnight previously she had got one.

'If I got a cameo blue one, I know everything would be OK,' she'd previously told us around the kitchen table, my brothers and I with our faces in bowls of pink Angel Delight. My dad trying to demonstrate restraint by not having any, at least not at the table.

The fun, bug-shaped cars, which came in funky colours and even had a kitsch little plant pot by the steering wheel to put a flower in, had promised joy. So my mum had worked and worked, now as a private psychologist, until she could afford one in her dream colour. The 90s white leather seats must've still smelt showroom-new.

She had hoped that this was the missing piece of her happiness jigsaw. Not her bouts of unhappiness, her lifelong problems with her sister, her isolation from friends living in the middle of nowhere, her stormy marriage and drinking too much, no, she liked to think that all that could be solved with a small piece of German engineering.

'It's alright Mum, it's alright,' my brothers said, on bent knees stroking her arms, hoping that psychological pain, just like a banged funny bone, could be rubbed better.

'I feel like driving into a tree at a hundred miles an hour,' she said.

She got up and paced over to the car-keys drawer.

Luckily I'd already thought of that. 'Where are my keys?' she shouted.

'Mum please just go to bed! You'll feel better in the morning,' I'd suggested.

I slipped my hands into my pyjama bottom pockets and comforted myself with the feeling of the fob in my palm.

She had marched up to her room and returned, eyes still filled with tears, holding an unfamiliar keyring. I didn't know she had a spare set. Those bloody Germans think of everything.

That day it was driving the car into a tree; the previous time it was throwing herself off the bridge beside our house. I loved my mum but also hated her for putting my little brothers through it all and potentially messing them up. Especially when sometimes these gestures felt like a pantomime, designed to create maximum drama, if only as a way of communicating something – but what, that she was unhappy? In what world did she think we didn't already know that?

At that moment my mum's work landline telephone rang in the hallway. She bypassed the front door and instead rushed over to answer the phone. We all knew to be quiet.

She wiped her eyes, cleared her throat like someone about to deliver a public announcement and picked up the receiver. '879 761 Abigail Waterhouse speaking, how can I help you?' she said in her singsong telephone voice as though she'd just wandered inside from picking apples.

As the parent wanting my mum's help with their child spoke down the line, my mum nodded and hummed, scribbling on the pad by the phone. By the end of the fifteen-minute call she was playfully twisting the phone's flex around in her free hand. All was well again.

'Thank you very much for calling . . . I'll look forward to meeting you and Duncan next week then . . . no problem at all . . . thank you thank you . . . bye now . . . bye bye.' She replaced the handset and walked upstairs to bed.

The next morning I went downstairs for breakfast where my dad was brewing coffee, the candles already lit. 'Morning!' he said. The worse the previous night, the breezier the morning's greeting.

My brothers and I, in our uniforms ready for the school bus, munched on our Coco Pops while reading the backs of the cereal packets as though the previous night had never happened. My parents drank their coffee together, discussing logistics and house jobs for my dad's day ahead as normal. Then my mum kissed us all on the top of our heads as she always did, retrieved the car keys I'd returned to their drawer and drove off to work in her shiny cameo blue Beetle.

'Helping others can be a defence from looking inwards,' Joseph says. It's true that the thing which always seemed to bring my mum back from the brink, more than booze or anything else, was seemingly being of use to others. 'It's the oldest trick in the book,' Joseph continues with a wry smile. 'As the saying goes; a cobbler always has the worst shoes.'

'So I hear you've got a girlfriend,' my mum says. Of course she knows already.

'Mum we've been for one drink.'

When my brother Gabe wasn't working silly hours at the Michelin-star restaurant, he ran a supper club from the Ikea table in his small Bethnal Green flat. His ethos of fine dining without the stuffiness was such a hit he's now going alone and opening his own premises called The Water House Project. And my parents have come down for the opening night.

They're staying in my room while I have the living-room sofa. Before they arrived Sam and I blitz-cleaned the flat and my parents strangely seem to have bought that we always have fresh bedsheets, use coasters and have a healthily stocked fridge. For breakfast this morning, instead of our usual sugary cereals we gave them croissants, orange juice and proper coffee to show how well we're doing in London. It's a slightly unnerving parallel with how my mum would spend hours making our house welcoming whenever visitors ventured out to our rural home. Although we haven't quite gone as far as putting a vase of wild flowers in the window.

'And Sam says you're seeing a therapist now. What on earth can you be talking about?' she asks. She finishes her flute of melon Bellini and instantly replaces it with another one.

'Um, we've spoken a bit about childhood.'

'But you had an idyllic childhood,' she shoots back, pure reflex.

I once saw on an Instagram meme that the secret to happiness is either to have had a happy childhood or a poor memory. Or is it that nostalgia has a funny habit of putting a rose tint on the past?

'It must be very boring for him,' my mum continues, 'I hope he's not just taking you for a ride.'

Unusually for a psychologist, my mum isn't a fan of long-term therapy. Which is a bit like a fireman who thinks that water is overrated.

'No it's helpful to talk, Mum. Like if I'm ever unhappy or something.'

'But you were such a happy little boy. If you're unhappy now it's certainly nothing to do with anything *we* did.'

I don't say anything.

She looks around at Gabe's impressive minimalist, Scandi-inspired premises; trendy East London foodies mooching around.

'Well we can't have been *that* bad as parents, as you boys have all done alright.'

I look at my dad and my other two brothers sitting at a table in the corner, marvelling at Gabe's achievement.

'I'm not saying you were bad, Mum. Therapy is fairly mainstream now, maybe you should try it?'

'Me and your dad once saw a couples therapist, but only for one session. She was useless. I knew more psychology than she did.'

'Well, maybe you should try again with someone else?'

'Please don't be nasty love. Not on Gabe's big day.'

And then she moves us on to more important stuff like where she's sourcing the Christmas turkey this year.

At one point a mingling woman with a small dog peeking out of her handbag moves dangerously close to us.

'Um, sweetheart let's move,' my mum says, her protective instinct kicking in. Despite her slim frame she's the sort of mother who would find that so-called hysterical strength to lift a two-tonne car off her trapped children if necessary. 'Or I can ask her to go? I'm sure dogs aren't supposed to be in here.'

I take a few deep breaths. After the initial fright, the spike in my heartbeat, and the quick prickle of sweat on my neck, I can already feel myself calming. 'I think I'm OK actually Mum.'

She raises her eyebrows until they nearly come off her head. Ever since I was little she's known me to cross the pavement even for chihuahuas.

'I've sort of been doing exposure therapy,' I explain. 'With a much bigger dog. So I think I'll be OK if she keeps a hold of it.'

My mum can't help but look impressed. 'Wow! Well I have to give it to him, maybe this Joseph character isn't completely useless.'

I don't have the heart to tell her.

17

TARIQ

Tariq flings his soaking rucksack to the ground and sits down, and after sniffing some dubious-looking stains, Tyson lowers himself into his usual spot of the threadbare carpet.

Outside cold, winter rain falls from the charcoal-grey sky in fat drops.

'Horrible day outside,' I jabber. Weather small talk to steady my nerves.

''Tis,' says Tariq, a man all too familiar with the elements. He declines my offer to dry his fingerless gloves on the radiator, perhaps knowing that they'll only get wet again later.

It's a bleak week towards the end of my second year as a psychiatrist. The sum total of my wisdom from time spent in the community: lots of people have complicated, shit lives. As a psychiatrist my role seems to be largely to tweak medicine doses, prescribe new ones, switch old ones around and wait to see what happens. A strange, unscientific human trial and error but one which to some is a validation of their very real suffering.

'Good to see you both,' I say to Tariq, nearly meaning it. I'm pleased to notice that in the presence of Tyson I'm no longer petrified, but one rung below. My heart rate must be a solid hundred beats per minute.

Just sit it out, Benji.

'How are you doing Tariq?'

'Same old,' he says.

I'm relieved to see him. I'd recently read about a rough sleeper who froze to death in the sub-zero temperatures, just metres from a luxury hotel.

'I thought about you the other day when we had that snow.'

'Yeah we got a shelter those nights,' he says and I'm encouraged that he's trying to avoid dying of hypothermia. 'It's not fair on Tyson when it's that cold,' he adds. 'You sure you're okay with him by the way? With your phobia thing?'

'I'll be OK if you don't let go of his chain,' I say as I massage the inside of my palm with my other thumb.

Accompanying the smell of wet dog is Tariq's usual cologne of alcohol.

'You can stroke him if you want?' Tariq says, no doubt trying to help me as a distraction from his own troubles.

'You'd make a good psychiatrist,' I say. 'But I'm OK thanks.'

He's right that if I could tolerate my holy-shit-what-the-hell-am-I-doing-worst-case-scenario of *touching* a dog, then maybe I'd be cured. Flooding therapy in action. That's presuming Tyson didn't gnaw a finger off.

'Let's talk about you Tariq,' I say, finally managing to prise my gaze away from Tyson. 'I know you said you don't want medication, which is fair enough. I've been thinking your mood might improve if you felt more purposeful. What do you read about in the library?'

Tariq ruffles his huge beard in thought. 'Philosophy. Social sciences. Psychiatry sometimes.'

'Nice subjects. I could help you get back into education if you were interested in working one day?'

'I'd quite like to be a social worker,' he says.

Patients often say this, often I suspect an attempt to right the wrongs of their own regrettable pasts in others. He looks into his lap, vulnerable, wondering if he has ideas above his station.

'I think you'd be an excellent social worker,' I say, and he raises his head a bit.

'I don't have any qualifications though. Maybe I could be one of those mentors at Alcoholics Anonymous.'

'You might need to get sober first.'

I detect a slight curvature of his lips. Subtle, but it's something. I'm also heartened that he isn't just fanaticising about suicide, but of a future life. In my notepad I write 'future-orientated thinking'.

'They're great things to aim for though. Why don't I ask our employment advisor to come to our next appointment together?' I ask casually, as if he's already agreed to continue seeing me.

'OK,' he says.

'Great. Also, you'll have more options if you stop drinking. Just something to think about. Should I write down where the addictions team are based?'

He scratches his huge crop of uncut and unwashed hair. 'Nah, you're alright.'

I sense that Tariq is at the so-called 'pre-contemplative' behavioural stage of change, in that he's not seriously considering it. The next available non-urgent clinic appointment is ages away but his suicidal feelings are long-standing, and he's never acted on them.

Predicting future risk over a period of months is hard because things happen. Psychiatrists are like emotionally drained and sleep-deprived weather reporters, who based on one brief glance at the sky must forecast if there'll be a thunderstorm over the coming months.

I hand him an appointment card. 'Do you think you'll be OK until we see each other again?'

Tariq smirks. 'I promise not to kill myself before then if that's what you mean. So don't worry, you won't get struck off.'

The line is barbed. Tariq has detected an unspoken reality to our meetings: that when I ask about suicidal (or homicidal) ideas, it's not purely out of benevolence. I know from Nafisa's early experience that if a patient dies, I could be summoned to a coroner's court to have my practice scrutinised in the dock by barristers and a judge, often with the patient's grieving family and journalists present too. Legal and professional eyebrows will be raised with everyone wondering whether the tragedy might have been prevented if my care had been different. Consequently, I often feel on edge, regarding my patients with suspicion, like unexploded bombs which might obliterate themselves, and me, at any moment. Medical education has drilled this into me too. In the practical exam which I'll soon have to sit, not asking about 'suicidal ideation' can mean automatic failure.

But some patients must see straight through our script, being asked the same generic questions from the manual *How Not to Get Struck Off for Dummies.*

I apologise for my robotic enquiry. It probably grated all the more since at times me and Tariq almost feel like mates. Not that doctors should ever treat their friends, as you risk losing your medical objectivity.

'Sorry, I sort of have to ask that question,' I add. 'But I imagine it must get annoying.'

'It's alright. But you don't need to worry about me. I've gotta stay around for this one haven't I boy?' He ruffles the underside of Tyson's chin. My patient's safety harness.

'Have a happy Christmas,' he says, standing up, and I remember not to say 'You too.'

'Thanks Tariq, you take care,' I say shaking his soggy gloved hand.

'Aren't you going to pat Tyson goodbye?' he says with a playful smile.

For my third date with Esther I've decide to cook her a meal at the flat. This morning I went to the supermarket for the ingredients.

In the drinks aisle I walked past the two-litre bottles of own-brand whisky, which is Tariq's poison, to source a vintage for Esther. A wine made from gooseberries.

Esther arrives her customary one hour late and I give her a tour of our flat including Sam's room-under-the-stairs. In the kitchen-cum-living-cum-dining room she opens the wine while I finish cooking.

'So tell me about your exes,' she says, leaning back into a chair at the kitchen table. 'Have you ever been in love before?'

'Esther has anyone ever told you you're quite intense?'

'Yeah, all the time. I take it as a compliment.' She laughs and peers over at the hob. 'Presumably you're aiming for intense not bland flavours in that food?'

'I suppose,' I say, stirring the carbonara sauce. Maybe I should add some tabasco?

'My sister is mellow like you actually. My mum says it's like she's on weed and I'm on speed. Well, have you?'

'I dunno really. I'm not really sure what love is.'

For Anton, love was the ultimate antidepressant. To Barbara it was flying thousands of miles away to doorstep a stranger in a wedding dress. To Paige, the absence of contact from her lover evoked unbearable, leg-slashing distress. To my parents, love is forgiveness.

'Alright Shakespeare,' she says, pouring the wine. 'Love is when someone makes you feel cuddled even when they aren't there. Oxytocin hormone basically.'

'That's a very Science Museum answer. Well, have you?' I ask. 'Cheers by the way.' We chink glasses.

'Cheers. Yeah, once with my first boyfriend. But he turned out to be a cheating fuckwit.' I can't imagine why anyone would ever be unfaithful to Esther, but I suppose Jay-Z did cheat on Beyoncé.

We both take a sip of the gooseberry wine and wince.

Thud.

'What's that?' Esther asks.

'Oh, it's the bodybuilding gym next door, but it shuts at 10 p.m. Then it'll be quiet until about 8 a.m . . .'

Crash.

'. . . although they're trying to make it twenty-four hours.'

Esther shakes her head then returns us to the matter at hand. 'The reason I'm asking is have you heard about these questions that make people fall in love?'

I turn around from the oven to face her. 'No.'

'Yeah, everyone at the Science Museum's been talking about them. It's like an intimacy enhancer which reveals deep secrets that would take a lifetime to discover naturally. Apparently if two people do all thirty-six questions it makes them fall in love.'

'Bollocks.'

She starts laughing. 'Benji you're so cynical. It was in a scientific journal and everything.'

'Esther I once read in a scientific journal that drinking aged urine cures depression.'

'Well, let's test it then! It'll be fun,' Esther says. 'The love thing, not the pee one.'

'What, me and you?'

'Yeah, like an experiment. To see if the results are reliable.'

I feel my hedgehog spikes bristling in defence, but I know that Joseph would want me to be more like an experimental guinea pig.

'OK I'll do it. Just to see if it works,' I say, taking a big gulp of wine. It grows on you.

She googles the article on her phone. 'Here it is. "The 36 Questions That Lead to Love". Printed in the *New York Times* too,' she says, nodding approvingly. 'OK Benji, get ready to fall in love with me.'

I abandon the food and we move to the sofa, light a candle and put on some music. The study's authors say vulnerability is the recipe for love but candlelight and Buena Vista Social Club can't hurt.

We take it in turns to answer the increasingly revealing questions. Vulnerable things we've never considered, let alone shared aloud. The theory is that by sucking intimate information from each other, it will bring us closer together, like that strand of spaghetti in *Lady and the Tramp*.

We admit to rehearsing what to say before phone calls. Imagine our dream dinner guests. We divulge what we'd change about how we were raised. We share our most treasured, embarrassing and terrible memories, although I soften the last one a bit.

'OK, Question 22,' Esther says. 'Share five positive characteristics about your partner. You describe me first.'

Esther is a no-nonsense eco-warrior who doesn't mind making noise for her causes (quite literally, she's in Extinction Rebellion's samba band).

'Erm passionate . . . fearless . . . colourful . . . fun . . . and beautiful,' I say.

'Thank you. Well for you I'd say intelligent . . . thoughtful . . . bearded . . . caring . . . humorous, sometimes.'

We discuss our mothers, but for some reason fathers escape any critique. Esther tells me that apparently like lots of Southeast Asian parents, her mum prefers talking about food rather than feelings.

'OK next question,' continues Esther. 'Do you have a secret hunch about how you will die?'

'Probably dog attack,' I say.

Next we share when we last cried in front of someone. We agree that there's nothing too serious to joke about. We share which family member's death we'll find the most disturbing. And which single item we'd save from a burning building (my revision cards).

The final task involves staring into each other's eyes for four minutes. It feels like a biological trick, like placing a newborn on a parent's skin so they bond. We swing sideways on the sofa so we're facing each other. For the first terrifying sixty seconds I fret about my breath, my facial expression and if we'll ever eat the pasta I've made. But then something shifts and I feel at ease. Like how people say when you're underwater the urge to come up for air disappears just before you drown.

Afterwards we kiss, because if you're not going to after gazing into someone's eyes for the time it takes to boil an egg, when are you?

Esther stands up and takes my hand. 'Let's go to your room. Actually no, let's go to the Harry Potter room!'

The Christmas work party this year has been organised by our receptionist Cheryl, who has decorated our table at Pizza Express with home-made crackers containing party hats and medical jokes. Apparently she's even researched some good conversation-starters.

Tonight Dr Cotton has made a surprise appearance too, donning a leather jacket. Christmas work dos are always paid for by the staff but Cheryl tells me it's an unspoken tradition here that the consultant pays for everyone's booze.

None of us are missing a free bar, least of all me.

This morning I had my end-of-year review with Sita. This time she didn't tell me I look too young to be a doctor. We discussed specialising in General Adult Psychiatry next year, when I'll be a registrar.

Despite not seeing me do much more than not fall off my chair in team meetings, Dr Cotton had written me an excellent report. Presumably so I wouldn't dob him in for being a shit supervisor.

No one had sent a reference from Daffodil Ward but Sita said that was probably because Dr Glick was off sick. Stress, apparently. I couldn't imagine such a thing. Sita kept calling her 'Iva' too. I'd never heard anyone call Dr Glick that. I admitted to finding her quite uncaring, which visibly surprised Sita. They'd trained together and apparently Dr Glick always stayed late, worked weekends, emailed patients' relatives, did anything she could to help. Ironically the last time I saw her was when she taught a session during lunchtime teaching entitled 'Surviving as a Consultant Psychiatrist', and had to end it prematurely because of an emergency on Daffodil Ward. Sita was drinking from her 'You Don't Have to be Mad to Work Here, We'll Teach You' mug. It didn't seem so funny now. I shrugged off the terrifying thought that Dr Glick maybe wasn't a monster but rather a product of the system.*

I focus on the good news that my library sessions with Nafisa have paid off and we've both now passed our written exams. And today is my last day working in the community before using up some annual leave over Christmas. Sita warned me that next year as a registrar I'll have more responsibility but at least I'll have a new consultant to guide me through it and surely they can't be as absent as Dr Cotton.

Soon the conversation in Pizza Express flows as easily as the Prosecco. I'm sitting either side of Rose and Darrell from our referrals meeting, whom I've never really spoken to before but who both seem lovely. It's nice that after the inevitable talking shop about how Darrell's ex-Broadmoor patient is actually really charming and gave him a Terry's Chocolate Orange, the conversation moves away from work and has a more personal feel. At

---

* Somewhat alarmingly, research suggests that over the course of a medical career, a doctor's empathy doesn't increase but *decreases*. Meh.

one point Cheryl addresses the whole table: 'So guys, how would *you* all top yourselves?'

I wonder if this is one of the conversation-starters she found online.

Given we consider the topic of suicide daily, just as a stock-broker might the FTSE 100, no one seems particularly uncomfortable talking on the subject. Even in our itchy Christmas jumpers, which were the mandatory dress code. So while in the background Mariah Carey sings about all the things she wants for Christmas, we go around the table describing how we'd kill ourselves.

Perhaps the most original choice comes from Dr Cotton. 'Cyanide capsules,' he says.

This is met with a chorus from the team of 'Mmm, good one.'

He justifies his choice of poison in some detail: how the fast-acting potassium cyanide found in Second World War spy-suicide pills inhibits oxygen absorption leading to rapid cell destruction, respiratory and cardiac arrest, with death not far behind. He says all this whilst dipping his dough balls in garlic butter, as LED lights flash on the nose of his Rudolf the reindeer tie.

The suited Christmas party within earshot of us, table reservation marked 'accountancy team', are unable to disguise their alarm. They probably don't realise that, contrary to popular belief, talking about suicide doesn't increase but *decreases* the likelihood that people will act on such impulses. So normalising its discussion is actually healthy. On my way to the toilet I seek to reassure our troubled-looking neighbours. 'Don't worry. We're mental health professionals!' I explain.

In the bathroom I now have the drunken confidence to check a text that has come in from Esther. I'm expecting her to say that the other night was a big mistake, too much gooseberry wine, but it's a photo from *her* Christmas party. The picture is of a smiling Esther, with a yellow sticky note attached to her fore-head which says 'Hermione Granger' and I actually blush.

I wobble back to our table grinning, just in time for my turn in Cheryl's macabre Christmas activity. As a thirtysomething male, statistically suicide would actually be the current bookies' favourite cause of my death, and that's before you've even fac-tored in things like me being a psychiatrist. And that annoying inner voice in my head which I seem to have inherited from my mum which sometimes goads me.

What are you waiting for?

For my answer, I plump for 'wrists in the bath', mainly because I love baths. Although if I ever did get to the point of ordering the vodka and razor blades, knowing my luck when the delivery arrived, they'd say that due to low stocks they'd had to make some substitutions. Next thing, I'd be sitting in a hot bath with my replacement waxing strips . . .

Afterwards, I feel like I know everyone better. And to bond with my team I didn't even have to visit Go Ape. And just like that the conversation has moved on.

'Why did Santa's helper see the doctor?' someone slurs, read-ing one of the cracker jokes. 'Because he had low elf-esteem!'

Everyone laughs far too hard.

Towards the end of the evening, once Cheryl's stopped hic-cupping, she clinks her glass with a knife. 'Right everyone, it's time for employee of the year award! Benji . . .'

I'm overcome with emotion as I turn to her.

'. . . when I announce the winner,' Cheryl continues, 'could you give them that gift bag under the tree behind you?'

The award goes to Darrell, presumably for managing to stay alive.

At eleven o'clock our waitress brings over the bill on a silver tray beneath some Mint Imperials. We've all eaten well and our mood is merry from all the free Italian beers and Prosecco. And all I have to pay for is my pizza and profiteroles.

Maybe it's the booze talking but as I watch Dr Cotton remove his card from his wallet, I feel a fondness for my aloof boss and a strange sadness that I won't be working with him again. I realise now that he's not measly with things like time or money, he's just really, really busy. He inspects the huge bill but to his credit barely flinches. We all look at him warmly, ready to show our gratitude. Cheryl even gives me a little wink from across the table.

'So is everyone happy to just pay for what they had?' he says.

On the night bus home I check my phone. After last year's fiasco with the Christmas cards bearing the wrong names, this year it seems our hospital trust has decided not to take any chances and has sent us all a Christmas email.

To: All staff
From: NHS Managers

Dear [Insert name here]

Seasons Greetings!
Thank you for all your hard work and to those of you working tirelessly over the festive period. We look forward to seeing you all in the new year.

With Very Best Wishes,
NHS Managers

DO NOT REPLY TO THIS EMAIL, IT WILL NOT BE READ

18

SEBASTIAN

'You're still happy to lead this one?' I say to George, standing outside our patient's front door.

George is the fresh-faced medical student who rocked up for his 'taster week' of psychiatry here at the crisis team.* He has bright red chubby cheeks and a shirt permanently untucked at the back. He reminds me of myself on medical-school placements, that same youthful ignorance too, no idea what he's getting himself into.

George was expecting to shadow a consultant but ours recently quit because he was summoned to the coroner's court so frequently they gave him his own car parking space. Since I'm now a registrar, and the team's most senior (and only) medical cover, George is shadowing me.

I enjoyed a nice Christmas up north where everything was reset and we all played happy families. Which was easy enough as somewhat confusingly we are generally a happy family now. Of course my mum still played her greatest hits about her retirement plans which are yet to materialise, and complained that my dad still hadn't finished our family home 'the mill'. And remained bemused that I can still find things to talk about in therapy with Joseph. I reminded her that a childhood spent trying to stop your parents from killing each other, or your mum from killing herself, isn't that 'idyllic' even if there are green hills and a tinkling stream. My mum had deflected it like a Ninja

---

* Crisis teams, or home treatment teams, as the name suggests see patients who are in extreme distress and therefore often at their residences.

batting away throwing stars, something about not ruining Christmas. She's a keen letter writer so afterwards on the train back down to London I wrote a long, thoughtful email to both my parents which they couldn't possibly swerve. I check my phone as George and I stop at our next patient's address. No reply yet.

We're facing the chrome-plated front door of a City worker called Sebastian who, according to the GP referral, is considering ending his life. We're in the nicer area of town: a florist is sandwiched between a chocolatier and a mini-Waitrose on the high street. Not your classic suicide hot spot.

Medical students need to learn a lot, and fast. Because of this, the accepted methodology in medical education is 'see one, do one, teach one' i.e. see brain surgery, do brain surgery, you're now qualified to teach brain surgery. Yesterday George observed me talking to patients, so today it's his turn.

'Sure,' says George, who raps enthusiastically at the front door. *Da-da-da-da-da—da-da.*

I'd personally only employ such a cheery NHS knock if I'd found the patient an organ donor, but I try not to judge George given some of my own mishaps as a medical student. Once on an A&E placement I told a gentleman with a round mass in his X-ray lung field that he probably had cancer (it was just a calcified nipple). Another time when taking blood from a healthy volunteer, I was so excited to finally hit the vein that afterwards I forgot to remove the tourniquet before the needle, so high-pressure blood sprayed everywhere, like in a Hammer horror, until the patient fainted. One urban myth goes that a keen-to-impress student at our medical school was once told to shave a male patient ahead of abdominal surgery and proudly wheeled him in having removed not only his chest and belly hair but also his beard.

When Sebastian doesn't answer his door I try a more sombre knock. Next I call the patient's mobile number on the GP's referral, but it goes straight to voicemail. Then I push a 'sorry we missed you' note through the letter box, the spring mechanism securing it half in, half out.

I establish the route to our next patient's address on Google maps and when I look up from my phone, George is pointing at the letter box. The note has vanished. I knock again and the door eventually opens.

'Hello?' says a thirtysomething man holding our note. He's tall, clean-shaven, conventionally handsome, and has the physique of a 5 a.m. gym-goer.

'Are you Sebastian?' I say, and he nods. 'Hi I'm Dr Waterhouse.' I've now stopped introducing myself as 'Benjamin one of the psychiatrists', partly because I'm the *only* psychiatrist in the team, and because as a relative senior now, I need to start acting the part. 'And this is George, a medical student. That note is from us. We're from the mental health crisis team.'

'Mental health?' he says, scratching his head before throwing his hands up in exaggerated bemusement. 'I suppose you'd better come in then.'

I enter, taking in the novelty for an NHS psychiatrist of visiting a palatial, no doubt multimillion-pound warehouse conversion.

'You have a beautiful apartment,' I say.

He smiles and gestures us to an L-shaped leather sofa. 'Coffee?' he says. 'I can't do anything in the morning without proper coffee.'

He flicks on the industrial machine on a marble worktop and starts playing Café Del Mar music through surround-sound Bose speakers. George and I admire the view through Sebastian's floor-to-ceiling windows. And is that an original Banksy on the wall?

'So what's this all about?' Sebastian says to me, coming over with a tray and some biscuits.

'Would it be OK if George led this discussion?'

'Of course, everyone has to learn somehow.'

'Thank you,' says George. 'How are you?'

'I'm fine,' Sebastian says straight away.

'Oh good,' says George and, relaxing, he picks up a Hobnob. 'So you're not still thinking about killing yourself then?' He asks this with his mouth half full, and I make a mental note to cover the rules of sensitive door-knocking *and* biscuit-eating later.

'Suicide? God no!' says Sebastian.

It wouldn't be the first time that due to an administrative error I'd been referred the wrong patient by the same name, or just the wrong patient altogether. Red-faced I fish out the GP referral from my bag. 'You are Sebastian Lloyd aren't you?'

He nods. Same address and date of birth too. 'Yes, that's me. How strange. Must be some sort of mix-up.'

'Well sorry to bother you,' says George, about to stand.

'Just a second,' I chip in. George still needs to learn not to always take a patient's word at face value. As if psychiatry wasn't hard enough without any objective markers to aid diagnosis, or any real cures, another potential complication is that of the unreliable narrator. 'Sebastian why might your GP have thought you're suicidal?'

'I can only think I maybe said something throwaway which she's misinterpreted.'

'Like?'

He hesitates. 'Like, um, when people joke that work is so busy it makes you want to blow your brains out. That kind of thing.'

George nods understandingly.

Sebastian seems quite guarded.

'Since we're here, would you mind if George practised asking you some questions anyway?'

'Sure,' says Sebastian politely. He's been brought up well.

George ploughs through the various parts of a structured psychiatric interview, but Sebastian reports an entirely uneventful history.

'And you work in the City, what's that like?' I interject. I glance at George, to let him know I'm taking this one.

'It's OK. Work hard, play hard. Crazy long hours though,' Sebastian says, laughing without clear reason. On the GP referral it said work stress had prompted Sebastian's disclosure.

He seems fine but is there a superficiality to his too-good-to-be-true answers? His painted-on smile? And what's a round-the-clock City banker doing at home at 9.30 a.m. on a Tuesday? 'The GP referral specifically said you'd been researching suicide methods online?' I probe.

Sebastian looks upwards as though rooting around for the memory. 'Um, no, can't say I remember that. I honestly think you've got the wrong chap here.'

'And in your job don't you usually work on Tuesdays?'

'I'm taking today off. Late one at the office last night, closed a big deal. I should probably be getting back to bed now actually.'

George rolls his eyes: it might be at my persisting with this clearly well gentleman when we have eight other genuine crises to see today. Or maybe it's just because we're now all out of biscuits.

'We'll leave you to rest then,' I say, getting up and heading towards the door. This coffee has gone right through me and we'll be away from the office all morning. 'Before we go could I use your toilet please?'

'Um. Well. Um . . .' Sebastian says, shifting uncomfortably. 'Yeah I suppose so.'

The minimalist bathroom is larger than my entire living space – a grand wet room with a free-standing bath in the middle and surrounded by huge, tropical plants.

After using the toilet I wash my hands with the bergamot hand gel and water from honest-to-God *actual* gold taps, drying them on an Egyptian cotton towel. I guess my suspicion is unfounded – what's Sebastian got to be depressed about anyway?

I turn to leave and only now from this angle do I notice it. It's in the back corner of the room, dangling from one of the steel girders which span the warehouse's high ceilings, tied at the end into a classic hangman's noose, a wooden stool just below it. The same electric-blue nylon rope my dad uses to pull felled trees on his tractor due to its high tensile strength.

In the hallway George has his shoes back on and the front door is already ajar. Sebastian won't make eye contact.

'Sebastian thanks for letting me use your bathroom. I think we need to have another chat don't we?'

He keeps looking at the floor. Then he closes the front door and walks back into the living room.

'I was googling ways to do it then finally decided upon the rope.' His voice has a different quality now.

'Go on,' I say, having taken control of the steering wheel.

'It's been up for about a week. I've put my neck inside a few times, just to see how it feels, you know? I was going to do it today. That's why I missed work. I'd just texted my family that I loved them and turned my phone off before you arrived.'

'You *were* going to do it today?' I say, picking up on his use of the past tense. 'Are you having second thoughts?'

'I don't know, maybe.'

'Sebastian can I ask, *why* do you want to end your life?'

He exhales loudly. 'Where to fucking start? You know when you have everything you could possibly want: big houses, luxury cars, beautiful women, but still feel . . . nothing?'

I nod as though I do.

Working in NHS psychiatry, I don't often come across City workers, but I've read stories of interns jumping from Canary Wharf skyscraper windows and CEOs calmly walking off the rooftop of cocktail bars holding flutes of champagne.

'And I've made some really bad deals recently. And what's it all for anyway?' he wonders.

'I hope we can help you think of some ways around this. In the short term I think that would be best done in a psychiatric hospital where you're safe.' He doesn't immediately tell me to fuck off, which is positive. 'It's probably best to have an ambulance take you to A&E. You'd get admitted more quickly that way.'

'No ambulance!,' he says firmly. 'I'll think about coming in, but not like that. People talk.' I'm encouraged that he's worrying about his reputation amongst curtain-twitching, busybody neighbours, which implies maybe he's expecting to see them again. 'I'll stay here and pack an overnight bag. I'll put my phone on so you can tell me where I need to go, it'll be close won't it?'

'Yes,' I overpromise, hoping to God there's a free hospital bed somewhere in London. 'And you're going to be safe?'

'You have my word.' He shakes my hand firmly and I wonder whether a gentleman's agreement is a valid defence against negligence in a coroner's court. I hand him a crisis-team leaflet containing some 'useful numbers' in case he needs us while he waits. 'And I'm sorry for lying to you guys,' he says. 'I'd just geared up to do it today and I didn't want to complicate things. I don't find it easy talking about, you know, this sort of thing.'

'Sebastian before we go, can I ask what's changed?' His work pressures, the emptiness of materialism or his lack of meaning haven't gone away and he could just be fobbing us off.

He pauses for a moment. 'Well, I know this sounds silly, and I've never really been religious, but I'm wondering if maybe you were both sent here for a reason.'

The only *reason* we're having this conversation is that Sebastian's GP sensed he was in danger and that I was desperate for a piss. But I don't burst Sebastian's divine bubble. On the rare occasion that a psychiatric patient thinks you might be their guardian angel, you've really got to take it.*

On the high street outside, George abandons the thread of professionalism he once had. 'Well that was a fucking close shave,' he says. He's right that if Sebastian had been our second or third visit of the day, his front door may never have been answered. 'Clever move pretending to need the toilet so you could suss out his flat,' he continues. 'Is that a recognised technique?'

I consider fibbing to seem more in command of this largely uncontrollable world than I am. But then I worry that this might set an unhelpful precedent, with George on home visits insisting that he urinate in every patient's bathroom thereafter.

'I honestly just needed a pee,' I tell him, the fluke of it still sinking in.

'Well, why did you bother taking away the rope?' he asks,

---

* God often takes the glory when things go right in medicine. But when things go wrong, He's never the one hauled up in front of the GMC.

looking at the bulge in my bag. 'He could always just do it another way.'

Sebastian had agreed to let me confiscate the ligature to join the assortment of weapons and other hazardous paraphernalia taken from patients' homes to later be destroyed. After a busy day, the contents of a mental health worker's bag can resemble a Cluedo murder-weapon inventory: ropes, knives, some have even seized pistols. Most social housing is bad enough though without us also taking away their lead piping.

We had stood on chairs untangling the rope together, like a family bringing down Christmas tree lights. I'd deposited it safely in my bag, then we'd left, walking straight past the bathroom cabinet full of potentially lethal medicines, and the steel chefs' knives in the kitchen, out on to the busy main road where double-decker buses hurtled past.

'People tend to decide upon a particular suicide method, and if that one is thwarted, they don't usually try something else straight away.'*

'*Usually*?' says George.

'Psychiatry is all "usuallys" and "probablys" and "hopefully nots". Predicting human behaviour isn't an exact science. We're just relying on clinical assessment, a gut feeling and sometimes a prayer. And that isn't always enough.'

'So how do you know he's not hanging himself now?' George asks.

'I don't. But because he let me use his bathroom I sensed part

---

* Suicidologists – yes that's a job – report that the single most effective suicide prevention strategy is to reduce the availability of deadly options which buys time for suicidal feelings to hopefully subside. Barriers at popular jumping sites. Non-toxic gas in ovens. Shop restrictions on paracetamol quantities. To use a more everyday example, it's a bit like when you're on a diet and empty the house of chocolate biscuits to avoid temptation.

of him, even if it was just 1%, didn't actually want to do it. That he hoped there could be another way. And just didn't know how to ask. A lot of people are like that.'

'Yeah people just have to ask for help don't they?' George says.

'Yes,' I say, even though this common sound bite – with the implication being that simply asking for help swings open the doors to timely, high-quality mental health support – is more rhetoric than reality.

I don't want to puncture George's idealism, at least not yet. I don't want to put him off psychiatry along with all the other medical students, given the speciality's chronic recruitment problems. So I don't mention that you also need to have the available resources and if they're limited, that a patient's level of need must meet the threshold to qualify. The grim reality is that lots of people summon the courage to 'ask for help' only to be told to 'go away and come back when you're worse'.*

I call the bed manager, who as luck would have it today is Brian.

'Hi Brian, it's Dr Waterhouse here,' I say trying to assert my authority. 'I was the junior on Daffodil Ward but I'm a registrar in the crisis team now.'

'Oh hiya Ben,' he says.

'I need a local bed for an informal admission please,' I say.

'No room at the inn,' Brian says. 'There are no free beds here or in the whole of London. Is it urgent?'

'Well, he had a noose hanging in his house so—'

---

* At its most farcical, some overstretched eating-disorder teams will reject referrals for new patients with anorexia nervosa because at 18 their BMI isn't *quite* low enough to qualify for treatment which they set at 17.5 or below. So, if the already dangerously underweight individual wants to be taken on, they must lose those extra pounds first. After which the focus will return to putting that weight straight back on again.

'OK leave it with me and I'll see if I can find something "out of area".'

At least my crisis-team job is also based in the Wellbeing Centre so I don't have to bother moving to another building. I now generally hot-desk in the crisis-team office, and when I need some privacy I've managed to retain my old windowless office. Cheryl on reception is another comforting constant, and when she isn't trying to save my light-starved cactus she's usually gossiping in hushed tones. On returning from my visits with George, just as we're walking past the main reception to the crisis-team office, Cheryl mouthes the C word to me.

Care Quality Commission (CQC) inspectors are to medicine what Ofsted is to education. They usually schedule their visits, which helpfully gives hospitals the necessary time to entirely change their practices. Revise their protocols. Complete patients' care plans. Draft in agency workers to give the illusion of full staffing. Then the CQC's assessments are boiled down to a single-word verdict, ranging from 'outstanding' to 'inadequate'.

Ahead of a planned CQC visit everyone is on their best behaviour and the place is mopped from top to bottom before you can say 'MRSA superbug'. It's the same routine that Sam and I performed just before our parents visited, when we transformed our flat into a totally different place. Just as my parents thought that the washing-up is never left for days in the sink or that we'd not go a week without bog roll, CQC inspectors must think that all NHS working environments are jolly, Febreeze-smelling, well-oiled machines.

Or at least they would, if they didn't occasionally, like today, come unannounced. Something that thankfully my parents are yet to do.

'Can we speak to your manager?' I overhear one of the two

corporately dressed individuals now ask Zara, the unlucky person who must have opened the door to them.

'Um, they're not in today.'

'Oh, when will they be back?' asks the woman.

'I'm not sure, we've not had a manager for several weeks actually.'

'Oh right. Well can we speak to the consultant then?'

'We don't have a consultant either. Our only medical cover is the new doctor, Benjamin.'

George looks up eagerly, like a dog that's heard *walkies*. I shoot him a glance and he dips his head back down. After a minute of cowering behind the monitor, I reason that I'd better turn on the computer. Then I call bed management for an update.

'Hi Brian, it's Dr Waterhouse here again.'

'Oh hiya Ben,' he says.

'Any joy with that bed?'

'Nah, still nothing in the whole country but I'm working on it. It may need to be a private bed.'

'I sort of told him it would be somewhere close. Any chance you could, um, make some room for him at Nightingale?'

We both know what I mean; odd that I'm now the one pushing to hurry along some hospital discharges.

'Leave it with me,' he says, putting down the phone.

'And you are?' I overhear one of the inspectors saying.

'I'm Zara, one of the regular Band 6 nurses.' Zara is London born and bred, experienced and a safe pair of hands. And being 'regular' not 'agency' means she's a long-term employee who knows the team and patients well.

'Well we'd like to ask you some questions then look around please.'

They have the charisma of a stapler. They perch on the side of a desk at the front of the office while the rest of us who are hot-desking stay glued to our chairs, hiding behind our computer monitors.

'So how is it working in this team?' they ask.

Beyond Zara's thin smile she looks like she's hanging on by a thread. 'It's great!' she says.

It's like the untruths I've told my parents about the job on my weekly Sunday calls: reporting that everything is fine, and omitting the insomnia, tension headaches and persistent feeling of dread. The things they don't mention at psychiatry career fairs. At least the CQC don't put pressure on me to bear grandchildren.

'First can you tell us who is the nominated first-aider round here?' the man asks through tight lips. The lines of his face are as angular as the clipboard he's holding.

'I think it's Lizzy isn't it?' says Zara.

'Based on our records,' the man says, studying his papers, 'it's . . . Miss Z. Mirza.'

'Me?!' exclaims Zara.

I'm now logged into the system and load our online patient database . . .

'OK never mind,' says the woman, who seems to be playing the good cop. 'Can you show us your local arson policy?'

Zara rustles through a grey filing cabinet by the whiteboard adorned with the names of patients on our caseload. 'Here!' she says.

The inspectors scan the document briefly, tick some box or other and add without looking up, 'And your national arson policy?'

How big do they think this potential fire will be?

'Um, what's the difference?' says Zara.

The inspectors look disturbed by this, as though they can't comprehend why, while trying to keep patients safe in our understaffed and leaderless team, we haven't found the time to revise the hundreds of local and national trust protocols.

And how different can they be? Does the local arson policy say not to burn things nearby but our national one says if you go to Middlesbrough, you can set fire to whatever the hell you like?

We all know that in the event of a fire in community teams, staff and patients simply exit to the fire assembly point and call 999. Psychiatric hospitals used to evacuate staff and patients outside too, but this was revised as most of the sectioned patients bolted as soon as they tasted freedom. So now hospital policy at places like Nightingale is just to shuffle everyone to a ward which isn't on fire.

'Sorry,' says Zara. 'There are just quite a few policies to keep on top of.'

I start typing my notes from this morning, whilst simultaneously eavesdropping on the CQC car crash playing out.

An anonymous young woman calls from a withheld number saying she's perched on a windowsill and is considering jumping. A social worker called Sid, with his best toothy smile, asks if I 'mind just taking it?' I nod but somehow in the transfer of the call, we lose her. Maybe he diverted it to the wrong phone or her mobile ran out of battery. I try not to think of any other explanations.

'Let's see your defibrillator and crash trolley,' the CQC woman is saying now.

'Oh easy,' says Zara, a little too enthusiastically, before scanning around the room in panic. Sid subtly points to the store cupboard and a moment later Zara returns from it carrying a bright green box.

'And you regularly check it?' says the man.

'Oh yes,' says Zara, brushing dust off the top.

The man peers at the paper inside, a list of dates and squiggles. 'It says here the medical equipment was last checked on . . . 2 October 2002.'

'It must mean 2012,' says Zara, bending over to look.

'No it definitely says 2002. So it's . . . nearly twenty years overdue.'

'I'd have been at school then,' Zara says quietly, she seems to be giving up.

The inspectors both scribble ferociously, and I wonder what Sebastian is up to right now.

A telephone referral comes through from a busy community consultant asking me to 'kindly' review a patient of his who wants to switch medications. This is definitely the consultant's responsibility, not mine, and I'm already drowning in work.

'Sorry we're the crisis team, and that doesn't sound like a crisis,' I announce. 'He doesn't meet our criteria so I can't accept that referral. Trust policy.'

The consultant abandons his pleasant manner. 'What's your name?'

When staff ask this it's rarely because they want to add you to their Christmas-card list. Maybe he wants to complain about me to my consultant boss. Good luck with that. I tell him and then the phone goes dead.

As I replace the handset I think of how close I came to leaving Sebastian's flat without using his bathroom.

'Right, stress and trauma policy. Don't worry about trying to look for it,' the woman is saying now. 'Just tell me, if you felt stressed after a long day what would you do?'

'Probably have a stiff drink,' says Zara. Which is not the right answer.

'I was thinking more, report it to your line manager?' says the woman.

'Oh yes I'd do that first too, *obviously*. If they weren't already off work with stress themselves.'

I imagine Sebastian hanging by the nylon blue noose.

The telephones keep ringing with new referrals or patients in crisis, and we rush in and out of the office trying to see them all in time. Thankfully the young woman from earlier called back and I'm trying to arrange a time for her to come in for an appointment.

All I can hear is the stone-faced inspector asking Zara to find a hot-desk cleaning rota or identify the food-hygiene officer.

I know accountability is important but part of me wants to scream, 'Can you seriously just fuck the fuck off and let us try and do our jobs?' George is looking at me funny and I realise that I'm glaring at them.

Eventually they go, and I call the bed manager for an update on Sebastian.

'Good news, I've found a bed!' Brian begins. 'The only problem is, it's in Durham.'

19

ROBIN

Esther has come up with lots of creative date ideas: a street-art tour, life drawing, a poetry slam, karaoke and salsa dancing. In the end, because of time, the lucky girl gets to help me revise for my practical exams.*

She's role-played a variety of potential 'patients'. The mute girl. The forgetful grandparent. The male flasher.† I must play the role of a model psychiatrist, diagnose her condition and propose a management plan. At least in these hypothetical worlds we're allowed to pretend that the drugs always work and that the patients won't wait years on NHS therapy waiting lists.

But it's hard to squeeze everything into a ten-minute interview. When Esther was playing 'Miss Dotty' with body dysmorphia who thought her eyes were too far apart, I forgot to ask if she was considering cosmetic surgery. If I had, I would have learnt that

---

* For my practical exam in psychiatry, just as at medical school, I have to enter an imaginary consultation room containing an examiner and a patient. After ten minutes a buzzer sounds and I'll move on to the next scenario. At medical school patients are procured for this strange speed date who have physical clues to their advanced, underlying ailments: clubbed fingers, big spleens, crackles on the lungs. These are called 'good signs' in medical education but they rarely spell happy news for the patient. So, if a doctor ever asks you to be a model for them, don't be too flattered. It means you're riddled with obvious medical disease.

† There are no physical 'signs' in psychiatry and managing genuinely unwell psychiatric patients for a day of exams would be organisationally ambitious. So psychiatry membership exams consist mainly of 'patients' played by frustrated thespians who like to show off their range, albeit to an audience of just two.

she was looking at YouTube videos on DIY surgery and that after our appointment she was heading to B&Q to get the tools.

Identifying such risks, and hospitalising the patient for their own safety if necessary, is key to passing psychiatric exams. I comforted myself then in the knowledge that 'Miss Dotty' was imaginary and tried to block out of my mind that the only thing preventing catastrophe in real life with Sebastian was my full bladder.

If being an Explainer at the Science Museum doesn't work out Esther could probably make a living on the simulated-patient circuit. She threw herself into her role with typical gusto, totally unfazed and improvising throughout.

On leaving the next morning I noticed that she'd left a tooth-brush in our bathroom.

I ring the doorbell to the red-bricked terraced house which has a neat front lawn and lace curtains in the windows. I'm alone again as George is off sick. I catch myself thinking, *He'd better be fucking sick.*

I wonder if the Sebastian incident spooked him. Or if it's because I snapped at him when he took a whole morning to see one fairly straightforward patient, leaving me with three extra to see. 'You've got to be quicker. Only ask the key questions!' I'd barked to him, as requests for emergency reviews piled up all around me. So much for me becoming the inspirational mentor I never had.

Yesterday I also received an email from the medical school saying that as there's no consultant supervision here, they're looking to move George to another placement. I resisted the temptation to ask if they could arrange a transfer for me too.

I do miss George. Plus it's safer working in pairs. But at least in his absence it's only with patients and during team meetings when I have to pretend that psychiatry, the NHS and me are all just fine.

When 'lone working', some take remote panic alarms, but they're expensive and battery-dependent. Plus, it doesn't help develop trust in a relationship if once inside someone's home, you ask if they'd mind you charging your panic alarm.

Others use code words, although they're not foolproof. Zara, the nurse in our team, told me about a time when she visited a patient who she usually got on well with. But on entering his house she quickly realised he'd relapsed. He was so paranoid he refused to let her leave, effectively taking her hostage. She persuaded him to let her call the office to supposedly check his medication doses. 'Hi I'm just at Dean's house, can you just fetch me the *red folder*?' she told the receptionist – 'red folder' being code for 'get the police here now!' But back then Cheryl on reception was quite new. 'Red folder, red folder, where is this red folder?' she said, rummaging around the shelves. She vaguely remembered something about code words and briefly considered calling the fire brigade. In the end Zara was fine, though, having escaped through a bathroom window.

I ring the bell again and eventually the patient's elderly mother opens the door, stooped over a Zimmer frame in a floral dress and with hair as white as a child's first tooth.

'Hello Mrs Butterfield, I'm Dr Waterhouse. Robin's community team haven't seen him in a while so they've asked me to come and check everything's OK?'

She shows me into the kitchen and gets out her best china, as some people still do for doctors. Above a two-bar electric heater on the mantlepiece are photos of Mrs Butterfield with her late husband, and their son Robin as a smiling young man. She offers me a Bakewell slice and after some chit-chat about the weather and local parking restrictions she updates me over tea. Robin is now forty, unemployed and single and they live together. They provide each other with company and though they aren't church-goers, she says they watch *Countdown* religiously.

Over the last week, though, Robin's begun venturing into the garden barefoot, stepping on the pine cones, digging something, before coming back in, muddying and bloodying her cream carpet. 'How do *you* get blood out of a carpet, Doctor?' she asks. I diplomatically tell her I have floorboards. She says Robin has stopped eating now too, so his trousers hang low. This coincides with her finding unopened packets of his medication in the bin.

A giant man bursts in. 'Who the hell are you?'

I rise from my chair, wondering if Cheryl remembers the 'red folder' routine. I smile innocently, trying to reassure myself as much as anyone that everything is fine. 'Hi Robin, sorry we haven't met. I'm Dr Waterhouse, a psychiatri—'

'Get . . . out!' he spits. My unshaken hand hangs in the air. His stay by his sides, trembling, as though fighting a powerful urge to knock my block off.

'I'm *fine*,' he says, head veins popping from his plum-coloured face.

I give up on the handshake. 'It's just that you've missed your appointments Robin. And I think your family have been wor-ried about you.' Trying not to implicate his mother directly is hard in a household of two.

He glares at Mrs Butterfield. 'You mean her? That fucking cow.'

Mrs Butterfield stares at her drink as though she's contemplat-ing diving into it.

'Your mum's just concerned that you don't seem quite yourself Robin. What are you digging in the garden?' I ask, as though I'm just a curious horticulturalist. He doesn't answer. Now for a harder question. 'And how's your medication?'

This gets his attention. 'I don't need medication. I don't have schizophrenia!' he says. Which is exactly the sort of thing some-one with schizophrenia would say. Or someone without it, which can make things quite confusing.

'I know you were in a psychiatric hospital for most of last year, what was that about?'

'Hay fever,' he says.

Daffodil Ward certainly wouldn't have helped with that.

'The doctor is just trying to help dear. Sit down and have a cuppa with us,' chips in Mrs Butterfield who, just like my grand-mother, seems to believe most things can be solved with hot beverages. It's a philosophy I'm now pretty open to myself.

'Good idea,' I say, 'and maybe some cake.'

'I get enough poison from that evil hag,' he snarls.

For a *Countdown* enthusiast, he calls his mother a surprising number of three-letter words.

I look at Mrs Butterfield for illumination. 'He thinks I'm a sorceress and that I'm poisoning his food,' she explains matter-of-factly. It seems odd that she left out this detail earlier in favour of offering me treats from Mr Kipling.

'Would *you* like to eat toxic metals Doctor?' Robin says now. The finger pointing at me has soil caked under the nail.

I'd recently taught George that when I first started, I naively behaved more like a barrister than a psychiatrist, trying to use evidence to change irrational minds. But by now I've reality-tested enough odd ideas, drunk 'spiked' water and eaten 'tampered' foodstuffs to know that delusions are by definition outside normal human reasoning. Eating the entire contents of Robin's fridge wouldn't change a thing. Psychosis always finds a loophole: 'she hasn't poisoned it yet', 'you've taken the antidote', or 'you're not human either', and so on.

'Robin what makes you think this is happening?'

'The taste. It's metallic, all of it. The bread . . . the ham . . .

even the fucking Fruit & Fibre.' Robin isn't talking about the fortified iron in cereals here. Likely, gustatory hallucinations – tasting something that isn't there. 'But don't worry,' Robin goes on, 'it won't be happening for much longer.'

Ambiguous statements like this need clarification. Like when a depressed patient telephones to say they're 'in a bad place', I need to check if they're suicidal or just visiting Peterborough. But before I can enquire, he lurches towards me, standing in that zone reserved for either kissing or fighting. 'Now get out!' he spits.

I don't much fancy deploying my now rusty self-defence techniques, and I have plenty of other patients to see. Plus I already have enough information to later trigger sectioning Robin under the Mental Health Act, the strange superpower I've now acquired as a registrar.

'Of course, I'll leave you in peace,' I say. Noticing the small TV in the corner I add, 'Besides, it'll soon be time for *Countdown*.'

'Ah,' interjects Mrs Butterfield as her hands struggle to replace the cake tin lid. 'He's stopped watching it actually Doctor. He says the words are direct messages from Satan. I don't know if that's relevant?'

Pretty bloody relevant.

'Well thank you for your hospitality,' I say, noticing Robin's flaring nostrils, 'Mrs Butterfield, would you kindly show me out?' I widen my eyes to her like captives do in films to signal to supermarket cashiers that they're in danger. But before she has time to reach for her Zimmer Robin barks 'I'll do it!'

Mrs Butterfield looks at me helplessly.

He escorts me to the front door and slams it behind me.

Back at the office I hastily complete the first of three forms required to begin the process of legally detaining Robin. Section papers are always Barbie-pink, maybe an idea from the PR team who first suggested naming psych wards after Disney characters.

At the end of my clinic I cycle to Nightingale Hospital to deliver Robin's section papers. At the Mental Health Act office an administrator in a coat and scarf is just locking up.

'Just put them in the tray,' she says, holding the door open and nodding to the desk.

As I exit Nightingale's long, familiar corridors I wonder how Blessing is doing. And if Dr Glick is back at work yet. I'm no longer the person I was when I first started here. Now I understand why the windows in the psychiatrists' offices don't open. In the staff car park I'd swear there are even more empty spaces.

My parents still haven't replied to my email and there's been a notable dip in communication. No weekly calls and unusually my mum hasn't rung to ask about my new placement. All I've had is a text saying that my uncle Thomas is unwell again and has developed the unshakable belief that an apocalypse is going to wipe out humankind leaving him the last person on earth. My dad doesn't know what to do for the best, so could I help? Another fucking referral. Stick it on the pile.

It's Sunday afternoon and since I'm not on-call nor speaking to my parents, I seize the opportunity to change my bedsheets for the first time this year. Once on Daffodil Ward a patient admitted to our occupational therapist that he only washed his every four months, something I could only dream of, and he was given extra support for 'activities of daily living'.

I'm stuck inside a fresh duvet cover, desperately trying to locate a corner, when my phone rings. On eventually escaping, like a crap Houdini, I see it's from a withheld number.

'Hello?' I say, still catching my breath.

'Hello I'm Dr Hart, an independent psychiatrist. Am I speaking with Benjamin Waterhouse?'

'Yes,' I say unsurely, hoping to fuck I've not misread the rota and actually *am* on-call this weekend. As I speak I pour the non-itchy washing powder into the tray and chuck in my dirty sheets.

'Benjamin some concerns have been expressed about your mental health so could we have a little chat.'

'What sort of concerns?' I say defensively, shutting the washing machine with a louder bang than I'd intended.

'This may be a stressful time but try to remain calm . . .'

There's an infuriating control to his voice which I recognise from somewhere, and for a horrible moment I wonder if it's an echo of my own professional lilt.

'Please can you not speak to me in that weird tone,' I say.

'What tone? Benjamin this is how I speak to all patients.'

'And colleagues, it seems. I'm not a patient, I'm a doctor.'

'Oh, I *see*,' he says, but his voice doesn't sound very believing.

I can hear the scratching sound of a fountain pen on paper as he feverishly writes all this down. I want to tell him to stop, but that probably sounds paranoid.

I wonder for a moment if this is an excellent April Fool's joke by Nafisa, but we're three months out.

'Yeah I'm sorry to waste your time but there's been a mistake because I'm actually a psychiatrist myself in charge of a whole mental health team.'

'*O-kay*,' he says. 'Is there anything else I should know about you Benjamin? Do you have any special powers, or can you mind-read?'

Seriously, this guy. 'Like I say, you've really got the wrong end of the stick here.'

'They're routine questions we ask all patient—'

'Are you listening to me?' I interrupt him. 'I've literally just told you I'm not a patient.'

This is also exactly what patients say. I worry that I'm just a few more wrong answers away from the men in white coats knocking at my door.

'Benjamin do you ever hear any voices when there's no one around?'

I'm really pissed off with this bloke now. 'Yes, I have a radio.'

'So you hear voices coming from the radio. What do they tell you?'

'Well this morning they told me to avoid the North Circular. I think it was an overturned lorry.'

He finally gets my sarcasm. 'Let's move on shall we. I gather you've been having problems with your mother.'

Has this referral come from . . . my therapist?

'Well, I mean. Yeah there are some long-standing issues, but nothing new, nothing serious.'

'What kind of thing?'

'Oh just the usual for firstborn sons who have supported their mums through volatile marriages. Probably too close. Overbearing to the point that I struggle to form romantic relationships myself, that kind of thing.'

'And you're planning to put an end to this . . . *dynamic*?' he says.

'Well, yeah I've moved 300 miles away. And I try to just speak to her once a week so—'

'Oh, that's odd. It says here that you live together. And, well, this is a sensitive question: do you ever think about harming her physically?'

'No!'

Is this referral from Joseph? During a recent session I'd told

him about a time long ago when my mum had been particularly malicious, following me into whichever room I tried to
escape to, shouting and screaming in my face incessantly with
her white-wine breath. And the fucked-up urge I'd had to hit
her to try and make her stop. But as I'd told Joseph, I'd left the
house and gone for a long walk. And having the impulse or
thought isn't the same as acting on it, is it? Joseph had even
framed it as a good thing, that I'd chosen a less destructive
option.

'OK last question from me Benjamin,' says Dr Hart. 'I gather
you've been receiving messages from the Devil via *Countdown?*'

My eyes widen to the size of snooker balls. Oh, I see what's
happened here! 'Um, I think I can explain,' I say, my voice now
calm. 'Which doctor referred me for this Mental Health Act
assessment?'

'I'm not at liberty to divulge that information. Now Benjamin, have you ever heard of "sectioning"?'

'Look mate,' I interrupt him, 'this is really stupid but I wrote
these section papers a few days ago for someone called Robin
Butterfield who thought his mum was poisoning him. I must've
accidentally mixed up the box for the patient's name and my
name, and accidentally sectioned myself.'

There's a long pause down the line, followed by a laugh. 'Don't
worry, it happens,' he eventually says. 'When I worked in geriatrics, I completed so many cremation forms, I once accidentally
handed one in confirming my own death.' He chuckles again.
'You'll probably need to re-refer this chap Robin, though.'

'Thanks, will do.'

'And don't worry, I'll make sure he doesn't lose his place in the
queue. He can have your slot.'

In my own words I tell him about the case, reducing Robin's
life to the most salient parts. Psychiatry Top Trumps.

Number of admissions: 9

Number of suicide attempts: 3

Previous episodes of violence: 1

Dose of antipsychotic medication: 20 mg but in reality 0 mg.

'Naughty Robin not taking his meds,' Dr Hart jokes. 'Is the property accessible?' I explain that Mrs Butterfield will let them in. 'Great. That saves us a locksmith then.'

Locksmiths sit ready in their white vans for the times when patients won't open the door. They use non-destructive methods such as decoders, lock picking or skeleton keys to gain entry. Plan B is to get the police to take the door off its hinges with a battering ram.

'Police presence necessary?' he asks.

'Afraid so,' I say, knowing that Robin won't willingly hop into the back of an ambulance. 'Roughly how long are we looking at, just so I can tell his mum?'

'About two weeks.'

'Two *weeks*? But this one's urgent.'

'I know, but they all are. We're really stretched at the moment. You know how it is. Did you tell Mrs Butterfield she can call the police if she ever feels in danger?'

'I didn't really get the chance.'

'Well I'm sure it'll be fine,' he says. Before hanging up he adds, 'Oh, and one more thing. Maybe speak to a therapist about that thing with your mother.'

Naturally the first call I make is to Mrs Butterfield to explain that it will be another fortnight until Robin's Mental Health Act assessment. The landline rings and rings until an answer-machine message plays. A friendly, male voice which is familiar but at the same time distant. 'Hello, sorry we've missed you. We're probably both in and have just lost the handset somewhere! Please leave a message and we'll call you back when we've found it!'

It's Robin's voice, although not the same Robin that believes his food is being poisoned and that the Devil is communicating to him through Rachel Riley's consonants and vowels. It's the other Robin who when well looks after his mum. If I could talk to answerphone Robin about his current self, I'm sure he'd agree that restarting his medication wasn't a bad idea. But I'm a few months late in catching him.

Lying in bed that night, an uncomfortable thought keeps re-igniting like those trick birthday candles you can never blow out.

I should have got her out with me.

20

THOMAS

The next day I call the Mental Health Act office for an update.

'Robin's on the board so we'll get to him as soon as possible . . . no, it won't be for a while yet. He was only referred recently . . . yes, with respect they're all urgent. Well, have you told her if she feels unsafe she can call the police?'

I decide to stop calling, sensing I come across as a green registrar who doesn't yet understand the system.

In our team meetings Zara, Sid and other members of our skeletal crisis team have already suggested that I stop telephoning, which could antagonise Robin or make him realise a Mental Health Act assessment is being organised and flee the property.

Alone in the staff kitchen afterwards Sid suggests I detach a bit and don't get as emotionally involved, if I want to last in this game. And he should know, given he's retiring soon. But it feels like a slippery slope between turning down the empathy dimmer, or going full Dr Glick-mode and hitting the 'off' switch. I thank Sid then call Mrs Butterfield's landline anyway and luckily she picks up. 'Oh Doctor, thank you for calling. Robin's going downhill, bless him.'

'Well please call the police if you feel unsafe?' I say.

'Yes, yes. I'll be fine. They want me here so I can open the door when they come to section him. I know he hates it in hospital but he's not coping. It's a terrible bind for a mother.'

And then she asks me something common for those in turmoil. A question which disregards my 'doctor' role and instead appeals to my humanness, with loved ones of my own. 'What would you do if it was your family?' she asks.

In the end my folks had decided that Thomas needed readmitting. He's in hospital now but isn't making much progress.

On Saturday Esther had wanted us to go on our first romantic break together and get the Eurostar for a night in Brussels. But this is a family emergency so instead she's coming up north with me to my uncle's psychiatric hospital. She's been badgering me to introduce her to my family after all.

On Friday night after work I join Esther on an Extinction Rebellion protest. We're very different, Esther and I, like yin and yang, but I like to think that between us we're a balanced team bringing different things to the party. For example, Esther is fun, passionate and socially conscious. And I make sure we're not late for things. And, as now, try to keep us out of prison.

'We need to get ourselves arrested to clog up the jails,' Esther is shouting at me above the chants of eco-protesters in Parliament Square. 'It's the only way to get this government to take the climate crisis seriously!'

She's told me before that mass arrest has successfully been implemented by Gandhi, the suffragettes and the civil-rights movement. I really want to get swept along by her altruism but I also can't shake the boring part of me that doesn't want to get struck off the medical register. Plus we're meant to be seeing Thomas tomorrow.

'I know. We'll attach ourselves to the front of Big Ben, to show that *time* is running out!' she says.

'Est, is it OK if we *don't* get arrested tonight? We're going up north tomorrow, remember.'

Esther scoffs; to her tomorrow may as well be next year, then she walks off into the crowd in search of superglue. Thankfully other, more organised activists have beaten us to it, have already been unattached from things, and thrown into the back of police vans. We're too late.

'Never mind Est,' I console her, as we walk back to our bikes. 'We can try and get arrested another time.'

Besides introducing her to members of my family, the other sign that things are getting serious between us is that I've bought us a 'Two Together' railcard. This means we're now bound together for the next year by the promise of 33% cheaper train travel, if nothing else.

'Please don't be late tomorrow, love. It would be really nice if for once it wasn't a mad rush. We're on the pre-booked 10 a.m. train so we have to get that one. So should we meet at King's Cross at 9.30 to get some nice breakfast things? Some coffees? Then we can get on in good time and read our books?'

'Sounds good. Stop stressing Benj, it'll be fine,' Esther says, giving me a kiss and cycling off to her flat.

As I cycle home I wonder if I should have helped her to mentally calculate that she'll need to leave her house at 9 a.m. latest to make our 9.30 a.m. rendezvous. But I push the thought to the back of mind, try to harness Esther's natural positivity, and reassure myself that, as she says, everything is going to be just fine.

It's 9.59 the next morning, and I'm in a position which is becoming increasingly familiar when catching trains with Esther, with one foot in the carriage and one on the platform to stop the doors from closing.

She'd texted me at 9.34 saying, 'Sorry I'm running a bit late but leaving now! x.'

At 9.52 she'd sent another text: 'Don't go without me! We can just hide in the toilets of the next one x.'

I'd been so looking forward to sitting in our pre-booked, forward-facing window seats in the Quiet Carriage. Enjoying the little bottles of orange juice I've now bought us from M&S, and the freshly baked *pains au chocolat* now sweating in my bag. Reading the paper or my revision cards. I'm less up for three hours trying to evade ticket inspectors in a bog that won't flush.

'This train is going now, sir,' the conductor tells me, not for the first time, as he blows his whistle. 'You need to decide, are you getting on, or getting off?'

I wonder if he thinks I'm just very indecisive.

The thing is that only a moment ago Esther texted me saying she was locking up her bike and to 'hold the train' for her.

'Sir I'm giving you one more warning, and after that I'm calling the British Transport Police to remove you.'

Why do all activities with Esther inevitably carry some risk of arrest?

The man's face is now nearly as red as his GNER uniform. And behind him I can see Esther weaving through the crowds in her purple dungarees and Dr Martens boots, with her backpack bobbing up and down as she runs.

The conductor turns around and we both watch as Esther runs round the corner and down Platform 4 towards us. Having established that the train isn't going without her, she stops jogging and walks the last few paces.

No sooner is she in the carriage than I board too, the doors close and almost instantly the train pulls away.

'Plenty of time!' Esther says throwing down her bag. She isn't even joking. She sits in our reserved seats and moves to the window to make room for me, but I just stand there.

'Benji, why are you looking at me like you want to kill me?'

My jaw is clenched. My fingernails digging into the pulps of my hands. I want to punch something, anything.

I snap out of it, turn and go to sit alone in another coach, my dramatic exit slightly ruined by the automatic doors which seem to have a life of their own.

I sit down and stare out of the window.

'Tickets please!' the jolly inspector says. 'All tickets please!'

I show him my tickets and railcard and explain with a faux-casual ignorance that Esther is just in another carriage, well aware that a requirement of the Two Together railcard is that, you know, you travel together. The National Rail T&Cs really need a subsection for relationship issues.

'Why aren't you sitting with her?' he asks.

'Right!' I say, coming to life, grateful for the opportunity to run my grievance past someone. 'So last night we agreed to meet at King's Cross at 9.30 a.m. . . .'

From the station me and Esther take an Uber to the hospital in silence.

When I worked in general medicine, during visiting hours the wards would bustle with loved ones bringing well-wishes, grapes and *Take a Break* magazines. Some relatives always pushed to come early, and others to stay late. That's not something we generally had to worry about working on Daffodil Ward. I seem to be one of only a few visitors on my uncle's ward too.

A nice nurse shows me to the Quiet Room, then brings Thomas through. 'And here's your coffee,' she says handing me a ceramic cup and saucer, a privilege not everyone enjoys. Then she leaves and closes the door.

As I pour granules from the sugar sachet into the brown liquid, Thomas watches as intently as a physicist adding uranium to a nuclear reactor. I ask him how he's doing, and midway through answering he says, 'Aren't you going to write this down? Don't proper psychiatrists take notes?'

I try to tell him I'm visiting as a loving relative not a professional, a point slightly undermined when I ask if he'd consider having the shock therapy his doctors are recommending since the drugs aren't working.

'Would it help you if I fried *your* brain?!' he screams at me. At this he thwacks the back of his head against the wall behind him. 'You've never had these medicines or electric shocks.' *Bang.* 'Psychiatrists never have to take them.' *Bang.*

Now probably isn't the time to tell Thomas that I have recently considered seeing my GP about starting something. A chemical fix to help me get out of bed, cope at work and to ease the dark thoughts. Quickly I slip my hand between Thomas's cranium and the wall. *Thump . . . thump . . . thump.*

I feel glad that Esther waited in the canteen.

The nurse who only just left, no doubt hearing the racket coming from what is supposed to be the Quiet Room, bursts in and on seeing Thomas's distress she asks me to leave. I prefer to think it's because visiting time is officially over, and not that I was making my uncle worse. So much for my family's fantasy that I'd somehow save the day.

I'm working nights this week so I'm resting in bed on Monday morning, reflecting on the weekend. Still no texts from Esther; maybe she's decided she doesn't want clinically mad in-laws. I haven't messaged her either as I'm still disturbed by the strength of the anger I felt on the train. It's all very well Joseph saying 'you are not your father' but he didn't feel his hand unconsciously forming a fist. And he wasn't the one seeing red, and visualising a Tarantino-esque quantity of Esther's blood sprayed across the train window.

Not wishing to dwell on this, I check my work inbox ahead of my looming shift tonight. Often HR will send panicked emails asking for agency workers, known as 'locums', to cover for rota gaps which exist due either to staff sickness or just because there aren't enough psychiatrists. Luckily no such emails have been sent, so some juniors and a consultant should be just a phone call away. But my eye is drawn to another email, sent late on the previous Friday afternoon, highlighted as of 'high importance'.

The email is regarding an unnamed forty-nine-year-old service user who was apparently living with his mother and awaiting a Mental Health Act assessment with a view to hospitalisation. The patient's NHS number and date of birth are included. Reportedly he is now wanted by police in relation to the murder of his mother. He could be armed and dangerous, we're told, so are advised to call 999 if he's seen and not to approach him. The 'not' is underlined.

Oh my God, poor Mrs Butterfield.

I jump out of bed and pull on some work clothes even though my shift doesn't start for another ten hours. It's pouring down outside so I decide not to cycle, or wait in the rain for the bus, and hail the welcoming golden light of a black cab.

'Beautiful day,' the cabbie jokes once I've squelched in and shut the door. His windscreen wipers beat frantically, syncing with my heartbeat. 'So where we goin'?'

I tell him the name of the main A&E in our trust where I can access the patient database. 'Righto,' he says pulling away instantly, the satnav in his head.

After several minutes, I can feel my mouth filling with bile, a harsh acidic tang at the back of my throat. I think I'm going to be sick. They'll put this in the tabloid headline: 'NEGLIGENT MURDEROUS DOCTOR ABANDONS OLD LADY THEN PUKES ALL OVER TAXI.' My body bristles with the need to be somewhere else. Maybe I should have cycled. Or walked. Or run.

'You a doctor then?' the cabbie says.

'A psychiatrist, yeah.'

'Go on then,' he says, one hand on the steering wheel. 'What am I thinkin'?'

There's one of those nodding Churchill dogs on his dashboard and his air freshener is the England flag. I want to say, 'You think they're coming over here, taking our jobs?' Then I bet he'd nod, seemingly impressed. But then I feel bad for stereotyping him. I'm not thinking clearly.

'I'm not at work now, mate,' I say trying to shut down the conversation. But I do clarify the difference between a psychiatrist and a psychic.

'So why do you want to work with loonies then?' he persists.

London is meant to be famous for people *not* speaking to you.

'Um, actually pal the correct term these days is "someone with mental health problems".'

He shakes his head and rolls his eyes. 'It's PC gone mad.'

'Not to be pedantic,' I correct him, 'but it's strictly "PC gone mentally ill".'

'So why do you want to work with *mentally ill* loonies then?'

Nearly.

This cab is so hot, sweat forming on my forehead, I may well hurl. I make it the final five minutes without regurgitating my Sugar Puffs and we pull up at the front entrance. Outside lush, cool air hits my face and I tip the friendly cabbie to curry favour with the gods. I sprint up the steps two at a time and flash my ID badge at the A&E security guard. For a moment I wonder if he looks at me funny, as if he's thinking, 'Oh *that's* the guy.' Then I enter.

Inside the bustling atrium of the emergency department I find a free computer at the doctors' station. The loading circle rotates painfully slowly before finally declaring 'Error detected with server – please try again later.' I don't have fucking time for later. I jiggle the wires at the back to no effect. Next, I give the computer some electroconvulsive treatment, switching it off and on again. Still no joy. Now out of ideas I ask the ward matron where I'll find a working computer, and she looks at me like I've asked her to prove Fermat's Last Theorem.

'I think there's a good one in minors,' a doctor says. They don't even look up, not entirely unusual, or do they also know that I'm the doctor who killed Mrs Butterfield?

I rush over to the calmer half of A&E reserved for minor injuries; a cleaner with a mop shakes her head as I skid past the yellow 'Warning – slippery floor' sign.

There's one free computer at the central nursing station. On my way to it a patient in the bay opposite me calls out for help and I walk straight past. 'That's classic Waterhouse,' I think, 'let 'em all die!'

I sit down at the computer, look at the login screen and in the stress of the moment go completely blank. Electronic patient records were tipped to revolutionise medicine by streamlining documentation and freeing up the time that staff wasted looking for paper notes, working pens or trying to decipher illegible doctors' handwriting. But they didn't factor in the time lost finding a computer that actually works or having to get past the login screen as you try to remember this month's unique password, with its requirement of two special characters, at least one number, some upper- and lower-case letters and which can't be like any of your passwords during the last three years.

After resetting my password to something I'll forget next time, I'm in. As I wait for Windows to load, I see Nafisa emerge from behind blue curtains. She scowls and comes over to me.

'Er, what the hell are you doing here?' she says.

She knows, everyone knows.

'Aren't you on nights tonight Benj?' she continues. 'I thought I was handing over to you at 9 p.m.'

'Nafs I've really fucked up,' I tell her. Of course, my time would come. My hands are shaking. 'Have you heard about this, um, "serious untoward incident"?'

'The homicide? Yeah it's so sad. Everyone's been talking about it.'

I *knew* that security guard, matron and doctor were looking at me funny.

'Beatrice was his psychiatrist you know?' Nafisa continues.

'What?!'

I think back to that first email.

Wait, is Robin *definitely* forty-nine?

'Yeah I feel so sorry for her. And the poor mum obviously—'

'Hold on a second Nafs, what's the name of the patient?'

'Um, Freddy something. It's all over the news, just look there. Why?'

My head flops back on the chair, and my whole body relaxes. But it's a fucked-up, perverse kind of relief that comes from knowing that someone *else* has died. And therefore my patient and his mother are probably safe.

I explain everything and Nafisa seeks to reassure me, before rushing off to see her next patient.

I need to be sure though. I turn back to the computer and enter the NHS number into the online database and sure enough it brings up a forty-nine-year-old patient called Freddy Todd. Then I read his notes so I know what it is I need to be 'aware of' if he presents during my night shift. But since that original email was sent last Friday, it seems the situation has already played out over the weekend.

It is documented that last Monday the patient's mother telephoned the crisis team asking about her son's Mental Health Act assessment. She was told that no date had yet been set. A few days later she called again, more distressed this time, asking for an update. Still no beds were available. When she called the following day she stressed that her son was deteriorating and that voices were now telling him to harm her. He hadn't actually assaulted her but the crisis team agreed to chase things up. Only a few hours later the patient's mother called again, begging for her son to be admitted. Now Freddy himself wanted hospitalising and expressed a concern that he may harm his mum. The case was escalated to the bed manager, and given the continued lack of any available NHS beds, the decision was made to look for and fund a bed in a private psychiatric hospital. The following day the patient's mother had been found dead at the property. Freddy was missing and wanted in connection with her murder. Given a manhunt was now on, the Mental Health Act assessment was no longer required, so it was cancelled.

Oh my fucking God.

Next, I browse the Internet and, just as Nafisa said, it's made national news.

Mental-illness-driven homicides have a funny habit of doing that and inevitably make the front pages, despite schizophrenia accounting for just 6% of murders[1] compared to 33% where alcohol or drug intoxication are present.[2]

The words seem to almost be swimming around the page, but I manage to decipher from the BBC website that on Friday police had launched a manhunt saying they were very concerned for Freddy and the public. Then over the weekend they found him in a park asking strangers if they'd seen his mother since she was exorcised of the Devil. He was seemingly unaware that he'd strangled her. The article says that he had been sectioned fourteen times previously. It is now in the public domain that days before her death, Freddy and his mother had both pleaded for him to be admitted to hospital.

I return to the database and now enter *my* patient's name. To my relief I read that only a few miles away Robin Butterfield *was* sectioned under the Mental Health Act and taken to hospital by ambulance. His medication has been restarted and he'll be discharged home once he's better, or as is increasingly the case 'better enough', so that his precious hospital bed can be used for the next patient in crisis.

I exhale the breath I feel like I've been holding in since opening that first email. On another day the outcomes of Freddy Todd and Robin Butterfield could easily have been reversed. But, down to luck as much as anything, it is Robin's psychiatrist, not Freddy's, me not Beatrice, who gets to telephone the next of kin to see how they are.

'Oh I'm OK,' Mrs Butterfield says down the line, her usual stoic self. 'I'm just relieved that Robin's safe and getting help. I was getting quite worried.'

'Well I'm glad you're OK and I'm sorry again about the wait,' I say, one finger in my ear to drown out the noise in A&E.

'Actually before you go, can I ask, Doctor, why does it always take so long to find a bed?'

I think about how to explain all this to Mrs Butterfield while staying professional and not showing my rage. 'I think it just boils down to the fact that people don't prioritise mental health as much as they do physical health,' I say.

She hums as if in agreement, says goodbye and puts down the phone.

Back at the flat I fall into bed and try to sleep before my night shift later, but obviously I can't.

Later on in court the judge expresses sadness over the preventable murder of Mrs Todd by her beloved son Freddy. They note the lack of available beds in the days before the tragedy and acknowledge the unenviable task for mental health workers to allocate the limited resources that are available.

Freddy Todd is deemed unfit to be tried for reasons of insanity and sent to a high-security forensic hospital for an unlimited time to receive treatment not punishment. Although arguably there's only one thing worse than brutally killing your mother while unwell, and that's having the harsh reality of your actions dawn on you once the fog of your psychosis has cleared.

21

BENJI

It isn't 7.11 p.m., 7.12 p.m. or even 7.13 p.m. It's 7.19 p.m. Nine minutes late for my usual 7.10 p.m. Monday appointment and I'm *still* in Joseph's waiting room. Why is everyone always late? And this after last week when Joseph forgot about my session entirely. Eventually the woman before me comes out and leaves.

Then Joseph saunters in to collect me with his hands in his pockets. 'Hi,' he says with his usual smile.

Fucking 'Hi'?

I lie down in silence for a good eight minutes until I realise this sulk has cost me nearly a tenner.

'It's still warm,' I eventually say, bubbling with rage.

'What is?'

'The couch, it's still warm from that woman.'

'Oh that's interesting. She's a trainee I supervise, so she was sat in that chair over there.'

I tilt my head back to look at the chair opposite Joseph's, the one I sat in the first time I met him. Am I losing my mind?

'Are you alright?' he asks. 'Is there something you're not saying? I'm sorry we overran . . . and for forgetting your session last week.'

It had been bloody annoying when after rushing out of work and cycling across London in the rain, his doorbell and mobile phone went unanswered. I'd stood on his doorstep getting drenched like a jilted lover. It's happened several times now. I'd really wanted to talk about the trip to see my uncle, or the recurring dream. Or Esther's lateness. But now it'll just look like I'm petty about timings.

'You can be mad at me you know,' he says.

I say nothing.

'You are not your father. This veneer of gentleness is just repressed aggression. You think you'll boil over, but you won't because you're getting help.'

This feels like another ridiculously optimistic proclamation, given how angry I felt on that train.

'You're trying to manage conflict differently, but you're over-compensating. Being able to communicate reasonable grievances verbally is healthy. All this "niceness". This "Benji" thing, you're infantilising yourself because you're scared of what you know grown men can do. But if you bottle everything up, then like a pressure cooker one day the danger is you'll explode over something innocuous. That's when you read about the loving husband who out of the blue kills his wife for forgetting to buy bananas.'

'These little theories of yours, Joseph,' I eventually say. 'How do I even know if they're correct?'

We who are Joseph's disciples, who pay him each week, are trusting him to be right, as he churns out blueprints for his concept of normal. But what if it later emerges that his world view is warped, that *he* is sick or demented or evil himself, and there's been a significant fault in the factory production line. Leaving us out in the world like those electrical appliances which need recalling because they could spontaneously combust at any moment?

'We don't know that I'm correct,' Joseph says. 'But I think you're holding back from me Ben.'

'Why the fuck do you call me Ben? I've told you a million times my name is Benji!'

'That's better Benji,' he says with a surprising calm. No explosion. No retaliation. No force.

Is he testing me?

I lie there in silence. 'I think maybe I know why I wanted to be a psychiatrist,' I say after a while.

'Go on,' Joseph says.

I peer up at him and he's shut his eyes like a philosopher in anticipation of hearing a new theory. He sometimes does this so he can focus on the words, but it can be hard to tell if he's deep in thought or having a mid-session nap. On at least one occasion he did actually fall asleep, later blaming it on a heavy meal. 'Benji I'm sorry for dozing off when you were talking about your anxiety that you're boring company,' he'd said.

'Well,' I begin, hoping to pass what feels like an end-of-year test, 'recently I've been thinking that I chose psychiatry so I could get the secret codes to fix my own family.'

Joseph nods as though there's a book of right answers somewhere. 'And how does that make you feel?'

'Well, it's depressing. After all of this training you realise psychiatrists aren't holding anything back. There are no secret codes.'

I close my eyes to stop the tears trying to form there. I've only used Joseph's Cash and Carry tissues once, and that was when I had a cold. Even with the couch's lumpy upholstery, I just want to sleep. But even if I could, despite my subsidised rate a therapy couch is more expensive by the hour than a bed at the Savoy.

'Where are you thinking?' Joseph asks after a period of silence.

'Nothing really. I'm so knackered. I just lie awake questioning every decision I've made. Did he seem quite guarded? Was she not telling me something? Why has so-and-so still not returned my call? Yeah, they're probably dead, I'll think.'

I catch my breath.

'It's always seat-of-my-underpants stuff. To admit a patient I have to fight for a bed and if I don't admit them, I worry whether they'll be safe. I just didn't think psychiatry was going to be like this.'

'Hmmm,' says Joseph. 'Not exactly *Frasier* is it?'

'Do you think I'm depressed?' I ask.

'No, I think you're an NHS psychiatrist.'

'Yeah maybe. But then why do I get these thoughts to . . .'

'To?'

'Oh I don't know. Just those annoying thoughts to kill myself. And that recurring dream.'

I'd woken up a few nights ago in a cold sweat, with that mixture of disorientation and dread. My heart racing after that same fucking car-park nightmare. Outside the sky was still black, lit up by the moonlight. When I looked at my phone, it was 3.14 a.m. I got up anyway.

Previously Joseph has put this down to what Freud called the 'death instinct'. He says at any one time we're caught between two opposing impulses of self-preservation and self-destruction.

'Joseph I know you can't catch mental illness like an infectious disease, but I do think you absorb something. When I worked in vascular surgery I had to wash my scrubs after every shift because they smelt of rotting flesh. You can guess what I smelt like when working in gastrointestinal medicine. But in psychiatry, what's passed in the air is people's pain. And you can't just rinse it off your clothes in the washing machine. It sticks to you.'

Joseph considers for a moment. 'Perhaps absorbing some pain is the cost of helping people,' he says.

Am I helping people though?

'You can't wash that stuff off in therapy either,' I continue, now too exhausted to care about Joseph's feelings. 'I sometimes think this process of trawling over the past is making me worse.'

I wonder if I've been brainwashed by the cult of psychoanalysis. Whenever I rabbit the 'it's good to talk' mantra to my brothers and suggest that they have therapy, they say, 'No thanks Benj, you're the only one of us who has it, and you're the most unhappy. No offence.'

My attempts to open up the conversation with my parents didn't exactly bear fruit either, and they still haven't acknowledged the email I sent them months ago.

'Joseph tell me, is psychoanalysis a science or just psychobabble mumbo-jumbo?'

'It's a science.'

'Oh good, so I will start feeling better one day?'

'Yes you will,' Joseph says, twice-tapping the oak legs of his easy chair. 'Touch wood.'

22

WHEN THINGS GO WRONG

'Which *side* of Suicide Bridge did they jump off?'

The question is all I can think about as I rush back to A&E just after 4 a.m. I don't remember when exactly I became like this; it happened gradually.

Inside A&E the rude matron I must've spoken to on the phone takes one look at me in my elbow-patched jacket, creased round-neck shirt, jeans and comfortable shoes and says, 'Psych?'

How do they always seem to know?

I nod.

'Sorry to interrupt your beauty sleep doctor. I'll ask him to jump off the *south* side of Suicide Bridge next time,' she says.

I force a smile for the matron who points me to a psychiatric side room.

Inside it a Registered Mental Health Nurse (RMN) is guarding the patient I usually only see during daylight hours.

He's hunched forward, his face bowed and his hands in those familiar fingerless gloves. Their grubbiness is contrasted against the pristine white bandages which are now bound around his left forearm and the sparkling plaster cast on his right wrist. He's quietly sobbing. In the air, that familiar odour of unwashed human and of whisky.

I just about manage to stop myself from yelling '*But you fucking promised?!*'

'Tariq, it's Benjamin. I'm on-call tonight. What's happened?' I say instead.

He doesn't even look up. He just keeps staring at the floor, whimpering and occasionally moaning. He's even dirtier than usual, but no more than anyone would be if they didn't have access to a shower and fell through a deep thicket of brambles.

The nurse shrugs her shoulders. 'He's been like this since I arrived. I can't get a word out of him.'

'Tariq you know you can talk to me,' I say.

He sniffs and tries to start a sentence. 'He's . . . he's . . .' he begins, and then he's sobbing again.

In my sleep-deprived state it takes me a while to register. Then a detail from the matron's original telephone referral comes back to me: '. . . *smells strongly of alcohol . . . saying he wants to die . . . best friend died yesterday*'.

Then I notice the empty space by Tariq's feet. And I realise Tyson's not here.

At the end of my night shift I go to the bathroom. I look in the mirror and reflected back at me is a pale, haunted-looking man I barely recognise.

On my phone there are still no messages from Esther but there is one from my parents: a wordless email with a link to an article about false-memory syndrome.

I hand over to the day-team doctors and join the bleary-eyed staff members in the hospital canteen for my post-night-shift ritual hot chocolate before I cycle home and try to sleep through the banging and crashing, as our steroid-infused neighbours pump metal.*

The jolly canteen lady greets us all warmly. 'Good morning love, how are you?'

---

* Everyone copes with night shifts differently. When I briefly worked in surgery, a colleague swore by taking a sleeping tablet before his twenty-minute drive home, so it would kick in thirty minutes later when his head hit the pillow. It was a solid plan until one day he unexpectedly hit traffic.

These small acts of geniality go a long way after an exhausting shift. Well, usually they do.

When I look at her now a part of me wants to snap and ask what she's so fucking cheerful for?

How am I?

I don't know what the fuck I'm doing.

I don't know what the fuck I'm doing.

I don't know what the fuck I'm doing.

I don't know what the fuck I'm doing.

'I'm good thanks,' I say. 'How are you?'

PART III

RECOVERY

noun: 1. a return to a normal state of health, mind, or strength. 2. the process of regaining control of something lost

23

CORONAVIRUS

When Sam gets in, he holds aloft a two-roll packet of toilet paper like it's the World Cup. 'I had to wrestle an elderly woman in Tesco for this,' he jokes, removing his face mask.

I continue playing *FIFA* while he washes his hands, which is the new normal. Then he flops on to the sofa and picks up a PlayStation control pad.

'Apparently in Italy the morgues are so full they're having to use ice rinks to store the bodies,' he says while we select teams. I say nothing. 'And in some hospitals here they're having to wear bin bags as PPE . . .'

'Uh huh.'

'Apparently the death count is now—'

'Fucking hell can you just concentrate on the game please!'

He obediently stares ahead at the screen as the pixellated players walk out on to the pitch. We both know you don't need to focus for this bit.

I could really do with speaking to Joseph but he hasn't worked out how to do sessions virtually yet.

'Have you done anything else today besides play *FIFA* Benj?'

'Yes! I've had baths. Three baths. I'm trying to relax, remember?'

After hearing that bubble baths are scientifically proven to reduce stress I went to Superdrug and bought six bottles. I've had three baths a day over the last fortnight I've been off, a prescription of forty-two long soaks. I'm not 100% sure they work, though.

Earlier today I poured in a good glug of the Radox 'Stress Relief' one, then I got in. It didn't seem to be doing much so I hopped out and added some of the 'Feel Blissful' one, thrashing it around with my hands to create the foam, and hopped back in again. Still nothing. Finally, now desperate, like a mad professor of bubble-bath alchemy, I added glug after glug of the top-shelf 'Sleeping Aromatherapy' one. I really need Radox to bring out one called 'Resilience' or 'Return to Work'.

'Also Benj, Mum keeps asking me how things are with you at work and I don't know what to say.'

'Tell her everything's fine. She'll hear what she wants to hear anyway. But she might be pleased to know that I'm talking to Esther again.'

Me and Esther had 'the talk' on the phone last week. We cleared the air about what had happened on our romantic weekend away. I said how her chronic lateness, even for things which I told her were important to me, made me angry. She voiced her grievances too; namely that I never tell her what I'm really thinking or talk about my family. I said I'd try to work on that. Also, she said I'd been 'acting weird' generally, detached, and was I cheating on her as I often had a bad excuse when she wanted to spend time together? She said she'd worked out that I tended to see them on Monday evenings, and that's when I came clean about my therapy sessions. 'This therapist, what's her name?' she asked suspiciously. I told her it was Joseph. She wasn't judgemental about me being in therapy, didn't think I was mad or messed up, or whatever. So when she asked how work was, I decided to fill her in on a few other things.

Several months ago, on getting home after the night shift when Tariq jumped from Suicide Bridge, I'd booked myself in for an emergency GP appointment. I deliberately didn't disclose on the form that I was a doctor, because I just wanted to be a patient.

'First name?' said the disinterested receptionist sitting behind the desk. You get a warmer welcome in Pret A Manger than some NHS services.

'Benjamin.'

'Surname?'

'Waterhouse.'

Having briefly worked in general practice as a junior doctor, I knew what she was doing: completing three boxes which ping through to the GP's computer beforehand. I was ready for her final question.

She slurped from a giant can of energy drink. 'Emergency reason you need to see the GP?' she said, louder than before.

'Um . . . depression,' I whispered.

She bashed the keyboard, spelling it aloud as she went 'D . . . E . . . P . . . R . . . E . . . S . . . how many S's are there in depression?' A patient behind me in the queue helpfully chipped in with 'two' as though we were playing Surgery Scrabble, and I went to sit down.

Like a train station's departure board, our names appeared on the waiting room's electronic screen. The receptionist seemed to have accidentally entered the 'reason-they're-seeing-the-GP' into the 'surname' box, and vice versa. Because up pinged: TREVOR HAEMORRHOIDS. Surprisingly, it was impeccably spelt. An old man, who had been standing beside a chair until then, shuffled to Room 2.

I alerted the receptionist of the error as I didn't much fancy being introduced to the waiting room as 'BENJAMIN DEPRESSION'.

When it was my turn I ended up in front of Dr Smith. 'How can I help?' he asked his computer.

I'd come because I wanted to try Prozac. Just something to boost my supposed serotonin factory settings and get me out of bed and into work every morning. Despite prescribing it hundreds of times, I'd only recently considered it for myself. Medications were for patients, not doctors.

Medics don't like being told the answers by patients, so I played dumb as I listed off my symptoms. It was all going fine until he enquired about work stress and asked me my occupation.

I'd better not tell him I'm a soldier.

Panicking I said 'Ski instructor.'

'Sounds fun,' Dr Smith said.

'Yeah, but I'm not enjoying it anymore. And sometimes I think about ending it.'

'Skiing?'

'No, erm . . .'

'Oh right.'

It was the first time I'd ever really admitted to having suicidal thoughts to anyone apart from Joseph. I've always had the impulsive, self-destructive thoughts of my mum. The ones which goad me to kill myself for as little as not receiving any texts.

Nobody likes you.

You're such a worthless piece of shit.

But there is one thing you could do!

All that crap. The thoughts always enter my head involuntarily, like unwanted guests, and I try not to let them get too comfortable or properly come inside. They just hover on the landing, still with their shoes on until I can kick them out. But they'd been forcing entry more frequently recently, and starting to sound more appealing, which in anyone else I'd probably think was depression.

They were still invading my sleep in nightmares too. Of course Joseph got excited about the symbolism of it all. The empty hospital staff car park I was trying to gas myself in. The callous corporate figure representing NHS management maybe, who only cared that any staff suffering wasn't public. We'd both chosen to overlook the fact that the dream might also have something to do with me maybe not wanting to be alive.

I knew I needed to pitch it just right with Dr Smith, though – depressed enough to get medication, but not so depressed that he referred me to my local mental health team. If only because it could be another name on my bulging caseload. Wouldn't that be a surreal moment, picking up a referral for myself?

'I don't think about ending it in a definite way,' I clarified, 'and I've never actually done anything.' I'd never placed that Tesco delivery or tried forcing the locked windows open. 'But just kind of, what's the point you know?'

Dr Smith looked at me for the first time. He had brown eyes. Tired ones. 'I do know,' he said. 'I tell you what, lots of things can cause tiredness, let's get some bloods.'

I didn't pull up my jumper sleeve immediately, but then worried I was overplaying the patient role to pretend I didn't know how doctors got blood. As though they just waited for women to menstruate or punched men on the nose.

'Roll up your sleeve, please,' he said. One 'sharp scratch' later he was clasping the blood samples that he hoped held the answer.

But the whole mystery of mental illness is its invisibility to medical investigations. I knew he was hoping to discover an 'organic' cause for my symptoms; something like anaemia or an underactive thyroid. Those things which can be so easily treated. I could really identify with his overwhelming desire to 'do' something.

He handed me a 'crisis team' leaflet, a bizarre moment, given I kept a bunch of them at the bottom of my bag.

'Good news!' Dr Smith told me down the telephone a few mornings later. 'You've just got low vitamin D. Collect this prescription, get some sun on your skin and you'll feel better in no time.'

I obediently took the vitamin D tablets as I continued dragging myself to work. I told Nafisa how the GP had prescribed me sunshine and she even invited me to join her and her fiancé on their Greek beach holiday. It was a generous offer but I thought a depressed friend on a romantic getaway could potentially be a mood killer. Plus I couldn't take annual leave anyway as that would leave the crisis team with no doctor at all. So, desperate, I tried bronzing myself under the UV tubes at 'Tanfastic' on the high street.

Two weeks later I found myself back in the GP waiting room. This time I noticed a poster about the prevalence of mental health problems, illustrated through hundreds of baked beans. 'One in four' it said, and about a quarter of the beans weren't orange. The colour they've chosen was remarkably similar to the NHS's iconic shade of blue.

I had a different GP this time called Dr Ali. She seemed kind, and at least she looked at me. It was quite hard convincing her I was depressed, sitting there with a full-body suntan. But at least she listened. My vitamin D levels were within normal range, she said, yet I told her the thoughts persisted.

'What's your job?' she asked, peering over her spectacles, with that textbook look of concern. Her computer monitor was turned away from us. Her room was warm and inviting. There was a happy-looking cheese plant in the corner.

I thought about the message to 'open up' like the can of baked beans in the poster. The idea that mental illness isn't something to be ashamed of, even for doctors. Maybe if I was going to get the chemical fix I was seeking, it was time for a different tactic. A dose of honesty.

'I'm a psychiatrist,' I apologised to my shoes.

'Jesus Christ,' she said. 'I'd better prescribe you some antidepressants.'

Back at home I stared at the prescription for 'fluoxetine 20 mg once a day'. The same thing that in my daily hurries I'd prescribed for patients, powerless to dramatically change their social circumstances: an all-weather, all-purpose psychological nurofen. I'd pictured myself taking it each morning then trudging into work like those Second World War soldiers plied with performance-enhancing amphetamines so they could march endlessly, stay awake for days and be numb to pain.

In the end, though, after much deliberating, I scrunched up the prescription and buried it at the bottom of our swing bin.

The 'chemical imbalance' theory of depression was first conceived by academic psychiatrists in the 1960s, and was enthusiastically promoted by Big Pharma, spoon-fed to the general public and swallowed whole, along with 70 million annual selective serotonin reuptake inhibitor (SSRI) antidepressant prescriptions issued in England. The theory helped antidepressants to become one of the most widely used class of drugs globally. Only now are psychiatrists admitting that there's no reliable evidence for the idea that depression is caused by low serotonin.[1] A bit late now, when 80–90% of society already believe it to be true.[2]

At work I'd become suspicious of this overly simplistic 'chemical imbalance' theory of depression. If this were the mechanism, akin to insulin in glucose control for diabetes, why did antidepressants not work in 30–50% of people? And why does the evidence only show them to marginally outperform a placebo sugar pill?[3] And that's forgetting the mountain of negative trials never published because they failed to show any benefit at all.*

I've long sensed, just as I had at the party with the woman in the fedora, that this reduction of depression to mere biology hugely underplays the messiness of life.

Undoubtedly, countless people have had their lives transformed by psychopharmacology. For some, antidepressants have been liberating and in some cases even lifesaving. But for others

* This is the medical equivalent of when someone uploads a video of themselves lobbing a basketball over their head and straight in the hoop, without also sharing the hundreds of other attempts when they missed. For more information on this and other biases, see Ben Goldacre's books *Bad Science* and *Bad Pharma*.

they do nothing at all, or psychologically numb pleasure too, cause grim side effects (alarmingly one of which is increased suicidality), unbearable withdrawal symptoms if they're stopped and can become an unhelpful distraction from the sociopolitical drivers of human misery.

If the current approach worked, I'd hardly mind. But medical anthropologists note that whilst outcomes in modern medicine are rapidly improving, there is only one speciality where they are getting *worse*. Psychiatry. A 500% rise in antidepressant prescribing since the 1980s means more people have access to these treatments than ever, yet far from what you might expect, suicide rates haven't decreased and society isn't getting less disabled but *more*.[4] Antidepressants are a blunt and imperfect tool and psychiatry is still awaiting its big penicillin moment.

I sensed my problem was less to do with defective brain chemistry and more linked with my environment. So, I applied for a career break. Just as with any break-up, I hadn't given the real reason on my application form. Instead of saying work was making me ill, I cited wanting to pursue creative interests. The classic 'it's not you, it's me' line. My application was swiftly rejected. Struggling with a mental illness, or a physical one, *is* considered a valid reason for a break, but I worried about it staying on my record. Oh, the irony.* Another always-approved reason, I learnt, is needing to provide childcare, but wanting a

---

* Stigma will truly have been beaten when people happily pretend to have a mental illness instead of a physical one, when pulling a sickie.

Employee (croaky voice): 'I'm not feeling well so I'm not coming into work today.'

Boss: 'No worries, it sounds like you've got a nasty cold.'

Employee (croaky voice still): 'No, it's not that. I've just been screaming into the darkness.'

Boss: 'Oh. Yeah, I heard that's going around.'

sabbatical doesn't feel like quite the right reason to bring a life into the world.*

I contested the decision and attended an appeals meeting with someone called Bob, who had the easy nature of a psychiatrist who'd retired from front-line work to take up an educational role. I fully expected him to query my 'resilience', the new buzz word going around which conveniently localises the problem within an individual rather than the broken system in which they work. But to my surprise he said, 'You *look* burnt out.'

It's a strange thing when what is famously so often hidden, starts to give you away. Worry lines have started to crease my face and people regularly like to inform me of how tired I look. Even a Jehovah's witness who recently rang our flat's buzzer retreated away from the front door saying: 'I'm so sorry sir, I'll leave you to rest.'

Bob said he'd try to overturn the decision for me and I instantly felt a sense of relief, closely followed by the shame of a deserter. I thanked him and apologised so profusely he said, 'Benjamin please don't apologise.' Then he flashed me a typed list of names from his clipboard and added, 'These are all the other doctors I'm seeing after you.'

With Bob's help the decision was overturned. The only slight problem was that it was approved from March 2020 onwards which happened to coincide with a global pandemic.

Sam and I continue playing our game of *FIFA* in awkward silence. I know there's plenty that he's not saying. I've been thinking about it all day myself.

I beat him, unsurprising given the hours I've put in recently,

---

* 'Daddy where do babies come from?' 'Well, sometimes when a mummy or a daddy doctor don't love their medical specialism very much . . .'

rippling the net with a last-minute winner. An overhead kick deep into extra time which I don't even celebrate.

'Aw fucking hell,' I say at the final whistle.

'What?'

I switch the TV off.

'I think I'm going to have to go back to work.'

'That might be good Benj. Although, are you sure you're ready? You have been taking a *lot* of baths.'

It's certainly annoying that after having fought so hard to get a break, this has happened only a fortnight later. But complaining about how a global pandemic hasn't come at a good time for me probably won't win me much sympathy.

'Oh fuck. Fuck fuck fuck.'

I've been manically checking the BBC news and getting updates from Nafisa about stuff the news outlets don't even know yet. She'd called me in tears after they'd had an emergency briefing about some psychiatrists being redeployed back to the general wards and a refresher on airway management for acutely unwell patients.

Coronavirus and its complications aren't just affecting people's lungs, but also their minds. The Royal College of Psychiatrists anticipate a 'tidal wave' of mental illness is just around the corner. Nafisa said 'this is our Third World War' and I knew it was bad as she didn't even mention that she's meant to be getting married next month.

Other doctors are coming out of retirement to help and there's even talk of fast-tracking medical students on to the wards to cope with demand. I imagine George with his rosy cheeks and out-of-bed hair inside a hazmat suit, absolutely shitting himself.

I know I have to return. I'd like to think it's a sense of duty pulling me back or maybe even heroism. But overwhelmingly it's survivor guilt. Also, if I ever have grandkids, I don't want them asking 'What were you doing during the great COVID-19 pandemic Grandad?' and my reply to be 'Um . . . I played a lot of *FIFA* lad.'

I want to jump up like a superhero, triumphant music in the background and announce, 'Yes there *is* a doctor in the house!'

But instead I just peel off my duvet, pick some Coco Pops out of my chest hair and scratch my arse. I locate my phone and with Sam smiling encouragingly, I find some energy from somewhere, adrenaline maybe or perhaps the Radox is kicking in. Then I call the HR department of the mental health trust I've only recently left, offering to work any vacant emergency on-call shifts.

'Thanks Benjamin. Could you do tonight?'

24

ANGUS

And so, only two weeks after leaving, I'm back.

It turns out that a pandemic ravaging the world is a helpful distraction from my own personal preoccupations, and I employ my mum's technique of throwing myself into the problems of others.

Some things are different from when I left. Intensive care is busier than usual but on psychiatric wards there's not much difference. Pre-pandemic they operated on average at above 100% capacity anyway. There's now a bit more PPE, but still not enough.

Eight hours into my first shift back, I know something is very wrong when I see Angus in the street without any shoes on. I had sensed it earlier in A&E, when he'd said that shortly after being furloughed, he'd discovered a coronavirus vaccine which would save the world. Which was even more remarkable given his qualifications aren't in virology but lorry driving.

I haven't thought what I'll do if I catch up with him, as he runs the wrong way down the middle of the road barefoot. What is it about losing your mind that means you so often mislay your footwear too?

Protocol for absconding patients, a medical euphemism for 'escaping', is to alert police who later visit their address and return them to hospital. But in his disturbed state I don't want Angus to reach home where he has young children.

Seated in our A&E bay I'd told Angus that, like his wife, I was worried about him and others, given he was still driving his empty lorry around the country having not slept for a week. For everyone's safety I'd said a compulsory admission to a psychiatric hospital would be for the best. Then he'd thrown a plastic chair at me. Which, if you're not medically trained, means 'no'. Then he fled, minus his shoes.

Security would usually have stopped him but they were busy restraining a family trying to be with a dying relative during his final, COVID-19-riddled, breaths. Amongst all the unknowns, while the necessary protocols are being drawn up, everyone is just doing what they can. And so, *I* pursued Angus.

He continues down the main road outside the hospital. Pre-lockdown, at 5 a.m. on a Saturday there would still be taxis, buses and some drunken revellers. Now it has an eery post-apocalyptic feel.

Exhausted, my own brain feels as together as vegetable soup. Abruptly Angus stops and turns around. From this angle I can really appreciate his size: eighteen stone of Scottish muscle, bone and fat. His freckled complexion is now red from the exertion or anger. What do I plan to do, exactly? Rugby-tackle him? And what if he charges at me? Almost on cue, he starts walking in my direction.

'Angus,' I say, catching my breath, 'should we go back and talk somewhere more private?' A stock phrase I've used before which make no sense now since we have London to ourselves.

'God, why is this man following me?' he says. His neck is cocked to the sky, his finger stabbing at the first clouds of the day. 'Tell me, is he trying to steal my cure?' A moment's pause. All is silent except for some early birds singing above us. He lowers his head, perplexed. Nothing.

It begins to rain lightly. 'The Lord is spitting on us,' Angus says.

His wife has caught us up now, stops him in his tracks, and gently caresses his hand, as though soothing a confused child after a nightmare. 'Gus you dafty, you're an atheist remember?' she says in her Scottish burr, gently taking him by the elbow. 'Let's get back on the pavement.'

Instead he takes a final step towards me. I don't need NHS self-defence training to know he isn't coming in for a cuddle. 'God,' he bellows heavenward, 'is this person trying to steal my *wife?*' I wait, my fate in the hands of the divine, or as psychiatrists call it, schizophrenia.

I presume he heard a 'yes' because at that moment he attacks me. Despite his sleep deprivation he has that manic, almost supernatural strength. In one kick he lifts me clean off my feet and on to my back, *Street Fighter*-style. Then he jumps on top of me, and she on top of him. We wrestle on the wet tarmac, grit in our elbows and faces close enough to smell each other's last meal. Moments before his pleading wife eventually manages to tear him off me, I remember thinking: 'I'm sure there was something I was supposed to remember this first night shift back. Oh yeah, that's it . . . social distancing.'

We manage to coax Angus back to A&E where he's left his belongings, and once there we wrestle him into a side room and slam the door. After the predictable banging, he turns his attention to singing the national anthem to the wall.

His wife turns to me. I've seen that look on her face before, on the faces of countless other shocked relatives. These aren't the scenes people envisage when they're slipping on wedding rings surrounded by flowers and friends; mentioning hereditary predispositions to psychosis doesn't tend to get the big laughs in best-man speeches. She probably thought 'in sickness and in health' meant making mugs of Lemsip for man flu, not tearing her beloved off a doctor. I've seen and heard about the pattern before, and not just with gardening-enthusiast Malcolm. After a few more episodes like this some partners find it unbearable and leave.

'I've never seen him like this,' she finally manages. She looks like the loneliest person in the world, standing only metres from her husband. 'He's usually so . . . quiet.'

'Haaappy and glooorious, loong to reign ooooover . . .'

'And he's a gentle giant usually.'

'I believe you,' I say, nursing my tarmac-grazed arm.

'Gooood saveeee ourrrrrr queennnnnnnn,' continues Angus.

'And I don't know why he's singing this,' she says, shaking her head.

'Well at least he's safe now,' I say.

At this reassurance, her forbearance ruptures, and a backlog of tears come. She hides her face with her hands, and I notice how the soft tissue of her wedding-ring finger has filled out around it over time. She'd need Fairy Liquid to get it off.

Nurses and I just stand there, the mandatory two metres apart. I pull a textbook facial expression of concern, the one which got me full 'empathy marks' in medical-school practical exams. But it's pointless, given I'm wearing a face mask. I've already broken social distancing rules once today by forming a human club sandwich in the road. If one of us has coronavirus, we probably all do now. What's another protocol breach?

I take a step forward and put a hand on her shoulder.

There's a subtle coronavirus undertone to most of the presentations I see as I endlessly plug gaps in the emergency rota, which arise daily as staff get sick or have to self-isolate.

There was the anxious young man so terrified of catching COVID-19 that he had panic attacks whenever someone sneezed. The girl with OCD who was so overwhelmed by germs that she washed her hands with bleach. The suicidal patient with depression who wanted to overdose on paracetamol but couldn't due to medication shortages. I know from Cheryl's texts that the Wellbeing Centre is being swamped with new community referrals too.

The stress of the pandemic is also visible online, and in the absence of authoritative information, and any scientific consensus, people are filling the gaps themselves. On Facebook, an old primary-school friend rants in capitals letters that COVID-19 is a social control plan activated by the government. Bill Gates is behind it. 'They' are going to put microchips in any future vaccines. And only Donald Trump can stop a Satanic-worshipping paedophile ring involving the global elite.

It's borderline madness, the paranoid fodder I'm more used to hearing on psychiatric wards. Maybe what distinguishes a conspiracy theory from a delusion is just if enough other people believe it.

As for me, I continue working, even if I can't quite put my finger on how I'm doing it. I don't feel great but that negative voice inside my head (not outside it) wouldn't be any kinder if I *wasn't* working. There's less time to worry if what I'm doing is helpful. And during emergencies, intervening seems more justified. Plus doctors can often find that extra gear during a crisis. It also helps that I'm free to stop accepting shifts at any time, and knowing that means that I never do. It's a sense of control I've never had previously, trapped in the remorseless hamster-wheel of a three-year-long registrar training contract.

Pre-pandemic I had once complained about my job to Esther, and in her typically blunt fashion she'd said, 'Have you ever thought about changing medical specialities? Maybe doing something like surgery. You might feel better if you were making more of a difference.'

My disillusionment in psychiatry, and my subsequent career break, partly stemmed from worrying that I wasn't helping anyone or that they didn't want it. But now the landscape has changed and new patients who have never before required mental health input are begging for support.

It probably also helps me that Esther and I have made up and decided to give things another go.

And with a killer virus on the loose, my ignored email is long forgotten, and I'm now talking to my parents again.

Several days later I get a call from the trust's 'Security Management Specialist Manager'.

'Benjamin I was sorry to hear about the incident on Friday night with Angus McLeod. Are you alright?'

'Yes I'm not too bad thanks,' I say.

'Are you sure?' the woman continues. 'It sounded quite nasty from the DATIX report. We wouldn't usually expect doctors to attempt to physically restrain patients, and certainly you're not required to follow them out on to the street, especially if they're agitated like that. We now offer staff therapy after these sorts of things.'

'No honestly I'm OK.' Then, trying to reassure her I add, 'I actually quite enjoyed the drama.' My face contorts at this irreversible overshare. I know it's too late; like when you press 'start' on a white wash, just as you spot a red sock through the washing machine's window.

'What did you *enjoy* about it?'

I decide against giving this stranger my life story, and instead just say, 'I dunno.'

'Well I think you *definitely* need therapy,' she says.

I'm getting sick of people telling me that. I take a deep breath. 'I've actually been having psychoanalysis for several years now,' I tell her. 'My therapist says I unconsciously do these things in adulthood to try and make up for the parental violence I couldn't stop as a child.'

'Oh,' she says, no room on her form for that. 'Well, you take care Benjamin. Bye bye.'

25

FEMI

'For those who don't know, Femi is a forty-five-year-old man with psychosis who believes he's a werewolf,' Reggie the nurse in charge tells us.

I've chosen to formally return to work as none of the emergency shifts I've endlessly filled officially count towards my registrar training. I can have that break in twelve months when this pandemic will surely be over. I'm running on NHS camaraderie, palpable national support and free 'feed the front line' sandwiches.

We're on the hospital's male Psychiatric Intensive Care Unit (PICU); because some minds need thorough care too. Hidden away in the bowels of the psychiatric hospital, it's where florid mental illness at its most disturbed and dangerous is housed.

Myself and members of the emergency response team are huddled inside the staff office which is like the large rectangular tank on Daffodil Ward, but with even thicker glass. It's like the viewing platform in an aquarium, from which to observe the more exotic, tropical fish on the other side. There's the usual din of a psych ward: occasional shouting and screaming, piercing alarms, the relentless banging and clanging of magnetic doors. And here, the previous trainee told me that these patients hit the glass harder, or fly-kick the door to get your attention.

Last night he gave me a frank handover on the phone: 'You think you've seen madness, and then you work on a PICU,' he said. 'The patients there are so unwell they generally have zero insight about their illnesses. So they're all on sections and because you often have to get medication into them through force, they hate you. But apart from that it's not a bad job.'

After hanging up I had put my new workplace address into Google Maps. The hospital was only a thirty-minute cycle away, but then I noticed its Google review score of 1.3. Unsurprising really, given the reviewers generally don't think they're unwell so understandably resent being locked up and forced to take medicines. This does shine through in some of the reviews.

Darren wrote: 'Modern-day torture house, evil staff, dangerous and highly ineffective treatments,' but curiously awarded it the full five stars.

There were other serious, specific allegations. Kwame wrote: 'These human rights abusers locked me up for six months and injected me with their poisonous medicines.' Underneath the hospital had responded: 'We are sorry our service did not meet your expectations.'

Kaleb seemed more easily pleased: 'My mother nearly died here. Free onsite parking.'

In the staff office Reggie continues briefing us: 'Femi went into seclusion yesterday after he attacked a nurse unprovoked, hospitalising them with a human bite. We'll go in and offer him some food, *not* the vegetarian option OK? Let's not make that mistake again. We'll try and give meds and get clinical observations and an ECG. Then the new doctor will talk to him,' he says looking in my direction. There's no getting away from the fact that he's talking about me.

At least I have a consultant on PICU: a warm Yorkshireman made from Teflon called Dr Tuke who dresses informally like me in a warm, woolly jumper, dark jeans and smartish trainers. Unofficially psychiatrists are allowed to wear trainers, maybe because their patients are more likely to chase after them. On arrival this morning he gave me the personal attack alarm now secured to my belt buckle. We'd agreed that he'd begin the morning ward round and I'd do the senior seclusion review. I jolted slightly at the reminder that I'm 'senior'.

'Anything else you think we should know, Doc?' Reggie says now.

'Um, about the werewolf thing. I am scared of dogs.'

'OK, well you can have full moons off,' Reggie says, which gets a laugh from the team. In this extreme environment, with such sick patients, there's clearly no time for my tame shit here, which I'll later discover actually helps me. I once heard about a study which found that depressed people tend to begin sentences with 'I' and as they recover their horizon broadens to instead focus on 'they'.

I quickly scour Femi's notes. He was admitted after neighbours complained of 'persistent howling' with his head out of the window. When doctors and police went to section him, he answered the door on all fours.

On admission it seems Femi was calm enough besides some growling in between sentences. He'd allowed the ward doctor to do a physical (he was hirsute, it was noted – but not overly so). He also consented to bloods but became angry when he wasn't allowed to drink the contents of the glass vials. He had leapt at the staff, gnashing his teeth centimetres from their jugulars, before sinking them into a nurse's arm in the struggle, puncturing his flesh and finally satisfying his desire for blood. Like a drunk diving under the pump after being refused a pint.

Someone has already entered Femi's diagnostic code – clinical lycanthropy – into the system. Before jumping to any conclusions I'd have liked to see what happens to the bitten nurse.

'Oh, and he's defecated on the floor,' adds Reggie, which seems a strange afterthought. 'So we need to clean that up too,' he says nodding to someone who's already holding a plastic bag and a damp cloth.

We drag our feet down the corridor getting suited into an armour of face masks, rubber gloves and tear-off aprons. Not my first choice of protective gear when going into battle with a werewolf. But I can't deny, a small part of me is strangely excited. As we apply our plastic pinnies on the move, they flap at the back like the capes of NHS superheroes. No one's sick of that yet.

A nurse is sitting by a robust, reinforced window. Video surveillance of the inside is transmitted to a computer monitor by her side. I peer at the CCTV screen which shows a small, curled, blob in the middle of the room highlighted against the bleached white floor. 'Is that the . . . ?' I say.

The nurse nods.

'How's he been this morning?' I ask.

'He's as good as gold when he's asleep,' she says with a tired smile.

I scan the seclusion pro forma beside her, completed in biro:

- Time seclusion began: '2.35 p.m yesterday'
- Has the patient been informed of the decision to seclude? 'Yes'
- Patient's views on seclusion: 'Fuck you all, I will fucking kill all of you, fuck you.'

It seems counterintuitive to wake a man who has promised to slay us, to give him a medicine that might make him not want to do so. But rules are rules and he's due a dose of medicine. Specifically, he's overdue it, having stopped taking his antipsychotic months ago. Strangely, I already feel less conflicted in this environment since the need for intervention seems more clear-cut. In the usual grey world of psychiatry, here the spectrum between sane and the other one feels closer to black and white. It's normal for us all to sometimes feel distractible, low, anxious, obsessive or sometimes paranoid, but even at pretentious dinner parties I don't imagine anyone ever muses, 'But aren't we *all* sometimes a bit like werewolves?'

The philosophy in PICU is to treat patients 'aggressively', sometimes with whopping doses of antipsychotics even above recommended safe limits in the *British National Formulary*, the UK pharmaceutical reference book. But hitting the psychosis hard, just like blasting a cancer in chemotherapy, means doing the same to the patient. And unlike in cancer treatment, in PICU the patient has rarely agreed to it.

'OK left arm, right arm, left leg, right leg, waist, feet,' Reggie says, assigning duties to his makeshift army. Everyone nods that they're happy with the body part they'll immobilise in the event of a scuffle. 'I'll take the head,' Reggie says nobly, which given Femi's biting history is surely the shortest of short straws.

Doctors are usually spared the physical work, partly in case it muddies the doctor–patient dynamic. Nurses have to try and establish a good therapeutic rapport *and* sometimes pin patients down, an impossible paradox, and unsurprisingly they bear the brunt of assaults on psychiatric wards.

'Femi, we've got some things for you,' Reggie utters through the intercom. 'Sit on the mattress with your back against the wall please. That's it.'

The reinforced door is swung open and the biggest nurses scurry in first like stormtroopers, with me at the back of the human shield. But no shots, fists, faeces or worse pelt us. Femi remains seated, perhaps still half asleep, his grubby bare feet hanging off the edge of the mattress.

Someone scoops up the poo into a bag with the casualness of a dog owner. Another removes his dinner tray, and the knife and fork look to have been used – progress. Someone else replaces it with a breakfast tray. These are the early peace offerings; hoping he'll agree to our requests to monitor his physical health, to take medicine and to stop taking chunks out of the staff.

'Good morning Femi,' I say stepping forward, like a cheery hotel manager just organising room service. Handshakes aren't advised in seclusion, even when there isn't a global pandemic, so instead I momentarily pull my mask down to reveal what I hope is a warm smile. 'I'm Benjamin, one of the senior doctors. Nice to meet you. I'm sorry there are so many of us.'

'You haven't brought enough. I have the strength of a hundred men. The government legally classify my body as a dangerous weapon because I could tear you all to shreds. Would you like me to show you?'

I know my predecessor was disturbed by the overt or looming threat of violence on PICU and would hide in the doctors' office when things kicked off. In contrast, in future when there's shouting or the shrieking alarm sounds, muscle memory will see me leap from my chair and rush over to try and mediate the disturbance. Old habits die hard, and I feel strangely at home here.

'No I'm OK thanks Femi. I was actually hoping we could agree to do a bit less fighting,' I say calmly.

Femi cocks his head back and howls. Then he uses his fingers to part his lips to show normal incisors, which he alleges are wolf fangs.

Given that challenging disturbed patients about their psychotic ideas is therapeutically fruitless and just antagonises them, some creative clinicians suggest tuning into a patient's 'psychotic wavelength'. Now seems as good a time as any to try.

'I don't think I've ever met a werewolf before. But werewolf or not, we can't tolerate biting ward staff. Is that OK?'

'Well if you give me the food I eat.'

From the notes I know Femi has solely been requesting raw meat. While NHS catering staff do try to accommodate most dietary requirements, he is having to make do with a paper plate of bacon and sausages.

'Well we've brought you a nice cooked breakfast, and that bacon looks a bit underdone,' I say. 'Would you let the nurses get your vital signs, temperature, oxygen saturation levels, things like that?'

'Don't worry – I'm immortal.'

'Right, well could we do it anyway? It's kind of hospital policy.'

A burly nurse wheels the trolley over and hugs Femi's arm with a blood-pressure cuff. Another puts an oxygen saturation probe on his finger and a third sticks a thermometer in his ear.

'I'm a 5,000-year-old werewolf. My oxygen saturation levels are 100%. My temperature is the same as molten lava,' Femi says.

A student nurse whose job it is to write down the results, looks at me, and I shake my head.

Someone calls out from the glowing lime-green monitor, 'BP 143/84. Heart rate 89. Resps 18. Temperature 37.1. Oxygen sats 100%.'

'Told you,' says Femi. Then he leaps up and snarls. 'Oh God, I can feel the beast coming on!'

The nurses hold their hands out, palms facing down to placate him. His eyes bulge from their orbits and I'm careful not to meet them, lowering my gaze in that way all animals know as submission.

'Femi I think everyone would feel calmer if you sit down again. Also, it's only the morning and I didn't think werewolves came out during daylight hours.'

'Is it?' he says looking around the room, disorientated.

He's been awake most of the night and there are no windows in here.

'Yeah look it's only just after 8 a.m.,' I say, showing him my watch.

'Oh,' he says surprised. Then he sits back down again.

The team and I collectively relax and thank God we're not working the night shift.

Now for the hard bit.

'Thanks Femi. Finally, we need to discuss your medicine. We've brought it in two forms, oral or an injection. It's nicer for everyone if you just swallow the tablets. Which would you prefer?' In psychiatry we pretend to respect autonomy, but the doctor's medicine usually ends up in the patient's bloodstream one way or another. Their only choice is how it gets there.

'Fuck you. I know it's poison to exterminate me.'

Friction during such exchanges often waxes and wanes, invisible forces controlling the tension just as the moon which Femi howls at pulls the tides in and out again. Up and down it goes, along with our collective blood pressures, usually falling with sufficient patience and verbal de-escalation. The problem is when a wave becomes a tsunami.

'It's honestly not Femi. It's medicine to help you think more clearly. And if you don't take the tablet I'm really sorry but we'll have to do it the other way.'

The emergency response team steady their footing. Reggie pulls the cuffs of his blue gloves higher up his wrists.

Optimistically I offer Femi the paper cup of tablets. He eyes them closely before slapping them away, then he charges at us, jaw wide open.

In the struggle Femi's arms and legs thrash around. I once heard about a psychiatric patient who somehow covered himself in butter as medicine time approached so he'd be harder to restrain. Femi hasn't gone so far as basting himself, but he's still a match for ten men if not quite one hundred, who chase after their allotted limb, though some improvisation and exchanges occur. When a right elbow jabs you hard in the eye socket it's hard to demur that you're meant to be on the feet. After a prolonged tussle of people grabbing what they can, every part of Femi's anatomy is pinned down by a different body, with me feebly standing above them, trying unsuccessfully to calm Femi with words. Next he's flipped over and secured on the mattress. Someone wriggles his trousers down and two needles, one containing antipsychotic and another a rapid tranquilliser, are plunged into the gluteal muscle of his backside. Disturbing animalistic grunts and screams spray from his mouth. The bulging whites of his eyes tell the fear of someone who genuinely believes he's being put down like a dog at the vet.

During such moments I can't help wondering if psychiatric hospitals are actually good for people's health. A ward patient once told me they weren't suicidal *until* they were incarcerated in a psychiatric hospital. Another terrified inpatient once asked me quite sincerely, 'Am I in hell?'

As Femi's struggling slowly subsides and the tortuous noises become softer, I wonder what the alternatives are. Let severely disturbed patients eat the staff for breakfast? Uncoil the asylum chains and dust off the straitjackets? Seclusion, physical restraint and enforced medication aren't a good arrangement, but are perhaps the least bad ones.

After roughly five minutes the powerful, high-dose medicines have been carried from Femi's buttocks through the bloodstream, until they marinade his brain.

Everything goes floppy, from his tongue to his toes, and he says he needs the toilet. One by one the emergency response team slowly release him and step back. Femi lurches to the adjoining toilet with no door and we hear him urinate in short, uncontrolled splashes, before he flops back on to the mattress.

'I'm really sorry about that Femi,' I say and I mean it. 'Maybe next time you could just swallow the tablets.'

A responsibility that weighs heavily on a psychiatrist's shoulders is when to terminate a seclusion. A patient showing regret about earlier violence and giving assurances about future pacifism, is probably safe to return to the main ward, a small degree of liberty restored. Lack of remorse, stated future threats or persistent psychotic symptoms relating to violence imply that seclusion should continue.

'Femi, do you feel bad about what happened to that nurse?'

His eyes are now sunken and lifeless. 'No,' he says groggily.

'And hypothetically speaking, if you came back on to the ward now, would you just be looking to keep a low profile or—'

'I'd kill everyone.'

Well, that's that then.

At lunchtime I'm rooting around the communal kitchen looking for a teabag and some milk when a member of staff comes in. 'Can I help you?' she says in a tone which translates as *what the hell do you think you're doing?*

'Hi, yeah I'm just trying to make a cup of tea before Dr Tuke's afternoon ward round. Is it a help-yourself thing here or can I pay into a kitty?'

'People have to bring their own.'

'Oh. Bloody coronavirus eh?'

'It's not that. We used to have a kitty and people were *supposed* to put £1 in every month, but it was always the same people paying, and the same people not paying,' she looks at me and I know which category she's putting me in. I think I'm more scared of this woman than I was of Femi.

I sometimes wonder why the NHS, as Europe's biggest employer, which splashes out hundreds of thousands of pounds on a single course of some cancer drugs, couldn't fork out for some milk, instant coffee and tea for its 1.3 million workforce.

Those 1p tea bags would surely pay for themselves through improved morale and productivity. And the time I'll waste trying to hack that combination padlock.

She enters the numbers to unlock it then opens a cupboard revealing tea, instant coffee and biscuits. She selects a teabag and I optimistically think it's for me, until she puts it into a mug which has a huge 'M' on the front, prohibiting the other letters of the alphabet from using it. Then she closes the cupboard, locks the padlock and mixes up the numbers again.

'May I?' the woman asks, pouring the hot water I've just boiled. Then from the fridge she adds a glug of milk from a brand-new two-litre bottle already bearing her name. I just stand there dumbly holding an empty mug which is probably somebody else's.

'Oh, sorry I should have said. There's a shop literally seven minutes away on the high street,' she tells me.

'Thanks,' I say, knowing I need to begin the ward round imminently. 'I'm Benjamin by the way, the new doctor.'

'Margaret, head of hospital care,' she says starting to walk out of the kitchen. 'I hope you enjoy working here, it's a really nice team.'

26

STARFISH

'Hello Joseph. You've got your camera off . . . the button at the bottom . . . that's it,' I say, flopping down on to my own bed after work. After getting his head around the technology, my Monday evening therapy now happens via Zoom to protect Joseph who is high-risk due to his age. One session he wasn't taking any chances, and even from the safety of his living room he kept his mask on for the entire Zoom consultation.

Since he's started 'working from home' during lockdown he's loosened the boundaries of the traditional psychoanalytic model. Today I can see he's sitting on his garden patio. Last week he really stretched the analogy of treatment as a journey and tried to give me therapy while driving to the supermarket.

'So how're you coping with the stress of the wards?' he asks, birdsong in the background.

I tell him about my baths and he chuckles. 'It sounds like 1950s bath therapy is coming back into fashion. Sleep any better?'

I explain that each night I now read the *British Medical Journal* in bed. Reading a meta-analysis comparing oral anticoagulation to low molecular weight heparin for thromboprophylaxis in patients undergoing non-cardiac surgery, actually works quite well for insomnia.

I did come across one quite interesting story in my backlog of issues that I somehow missed. That of a consultant psychiatrist who worked for twenty-two years, until she was found to be a fake doctor. You might expect that her poor outcomes would be an obvious red flag, but despite having zero qualifications, no concerns were flagged up about Zholia Alemi's clinical expertise. On the contrary, during her trial she was said to have given 'very reasonable' care. Suspicions were only raised when she forged an elderly patient's will to become the beneficiary of their estate.

'It's crazy right. *Twenty-two years,*' I ponder aloud to Joseph. 'How the hell could she do that?'

Joseph takes my moral question surprisingly literally. 'You can get white coats from fancy-dress shops,' he says. 'That, combined with some dodgy credentials and an inherent trust of doctors, I suppose.* And I guess if any patients did raise suspicions about their psychiatrist being a fake, they'd just have their meds increased.'†

Joseph laughs at his own dark joke and sneaks a sip of iced water. Or is it a gin and tonic? 'It makes you wonder how rigorous the science of psychiatry really is,' he says.

In several years, I'll be a consultant, yet I still feel so uninformed. That bloody Dunning–Kruger effect again; the more I know the less I feel like I know. But also there clearly *is* still much to discover if an impostor can bypass five years at medical school, two as a junior doctor, and six in speciality psychiatry training without anyone even noticing.

'Well, yeah, when you can't tell a consultant psychiatrist from

---

* A quick Google search revealed the story of a bogus obstetrician in Melbourne who told desperate IVF couples they were pregnant when they weren't, and a sham surgeon in California who was only rumbled after he printed a giant image of his face on to his white coat (which was considered too narcissistic even for a surgeon).

† On PICU a sick patient once reported seeing little animals scurrying around his room at night. Dr Tuke wrote him up for another antipsychotic to target these visual hallucinations. Then, during a night shift I saw the mice myself. I crossed off his new prescription and instead emailed the pest controllers.

a con artist it does make me wonder how necessary all this fancy training is,' I concede.

'It's the same in psychotherapy. We use showy words because science demands that there's a common language. And it gives us gravitas. But research shows the single biggest determinant of whether a patient improves isn't the therapist's level of qualification, the years of experience or the type of therapy.'

'What is it?'

Joseph leaves one of his trademark dramatic pauses: '. . .The quality of the therapist–patient relationship.'[1]

'Wow,' I say, the simple power of this slowly sinking in.

'Are you mentioning all this because you're thinking about leaving?' he asks.

I've endlessly complained to Joseph about how conflicted I am. And sometimes psychiatry's problems seem too big for individuals. Even if I try to practise more ethically, whatever that looks like, I'd still feel the same hopelessness I get when washing-up my recycling to combat the climate crisis.

Or maybe it's too convenient to blame my troubled profession for my melancholy; haven't I *always* really struggled to be happy?*

Psychiatry is certainly problematic, but it faces some unique challenges compared to other specialities.

'I don't think I'll ever quit,' I say to Joseph. 'I like it. I mean often I don't, but you know what I mean. I just want it to be . . . better. Sometimes you wonder if the government is deliberately

---

* Research suggests that even at medical school those students wishing to specialise in psychiatry are *already* more depressed than their contemporaries considering other specialities. So the profession inherently attracts troubled souls, and spending their working lives around human misery doesn't help much either. Maybe the logic is that if you're going to end up on a psych ward one way or another, you may as well get paid for it.

trying to destroy the NHS too. But I don't think you can improve anything by abandoning it, can you?'

'That's true.'

I can usually overcome my defeatism, perhaps in the hope that some day things will improve. It's this same ideology that's seen my mum and dad show commitment to their marriage despite the bumpy times. That stickability is something I should probably acknowledge on our next Sunday phone call. They've taught me not to walk away.

'But the reality is different to what I was expecting. You know in my medical-school interview someone on the panel asked me how I'd like to change the world?'

Joseph laughs. 'They obviously had a God complex. You can't save everyone, but that's no reason to give up. Have I told you the starfish fable?'

'No, I don't think so.'

Joseph quenches his thirst again before starting. 'So an old man is walking along a beach littered with starfish washed ashore from a high tide when he comes across a boy throwing them back into the ocean. The man asks what he's doing and the boy tells him "I'm saving these starfish." The old man chuckles and says, "Son, there are thousands of starfish and only one of you. What difference can you make?" The boy picks up a starfish, gently tosses it into the water and says, "I made a difference to that one."'

27

ESCAPING PSYCHIATRY

It's the Friday before the bank holiday weekend, and due to a heatwave the ward is a jungle-like 33°C, with its non-opening windows and impossible-to-turn-off NHS radiators on full blast. When it gets like this some dusty old fans will emerge to helpfully push the hot air around a bit.

I find a topless Femi standing gazing out of his bedroom window at a red-brick wall. His uninspiring view of the building next to us is framed by fire-resistant curtains on a magnetic rail which collapse if you merely hang your hopes of discharge on them.

Now several months into his treatment with psychotropic drugs, Femi's delusional ideas about wolf-transformation have vanished, and since he returned to the open ward he hasn't demanded a carnivorous diet. During a recent cookery group with our occupational therapist he made a mushroom pizza which he shared with everyone. Although the aliveness of his eyes has now been replaced with a dullness.

I poke my head around his door and briefly lower my mask to show what again I hope is a warm smile. 'Femi, are you free? For your ward round I mean. I'm doing it today as Dr Tuke is at a training day.'

'Can we just talk here in my cell?' he says.

'This isn't your cell, it's your bedroom.'

He huffs. 'So when am I getting out of here?' he asks, looking longingly back out of his window at the brick wall.

'Soon. Once we've swapped over your risperidone.'

After finally finding a medicine that successfully shifted Femi's delusions, there's a catch. Side effects.

'I still feel like I'm turning into a woman. My dick doesn't work and I'm growing man-boobs.' He sits down on his bed to deliver the worst news. 'And *milk* is coming out of my nipples.'

'I'm really sorry Femi, yes that can happen.' Femi's current antipsychotic risperidone can elevate prolactin hormone to levels normally only seen in pregnant women or new mothers.

We discuss the alternatives and their common side effects. Olanzapine (lethargy, weight gain, diabetes, heart disease). Quetiapine (the same). Aripiprazole (an inner restlessness called 'akathisia' that's so unpleasant some patients take their own lives). Older-generation antipsychotics like Clopixol (odd movements like rocking, shaking, ticking, irreversible mouth and tongue spasms). Or clozapine, the top-shelf antipsychotic with the strongest evidence base (potentially fatal heart inflammation, deadly lowering of the body's white cells which fight infection, and severe constipation leading to bowel perforation which is what kills those who take it most frequently).

It's no wonder that patients aren't always reassured when psychiatrists say they're excellent medicines and not to worry.

'I don't want to take any of those dirty drugs,' he says.

'Femi unfortunately the gold-standard treatment in this country is antipsychotics.'*

---

* An uncomfortable truth is that in terms of outcomes, people with serious mental illness actually fare *better* in the developing world (where there is less availability of drugs and stronger family ties) than they do here (WHO, 1973). With this in mind, 'Open Dialogue' is a potentially revolutionary Finnish model of care where patients can choose 'drug-free' treatment. Medication is optional and more time, curiosity and non-pharmacological resources are invested in patients. Remarkably under this less coercive model, 76% of 'Open Dialogue' patients (only a third of whom have used antipsychotics) return to work or study within five years (J. Seikkula et al., 2006). In the UK (where medication is the mainstay of treatment) only 8% of people with schizophrenia are in employment.

'I'd love to see you take these fucking pills,' he says. It's something my uncle Thomas has invited me to do before too.

I once considered asking Pharmacy for the ward's out-of-date antipsychotics which would only be destroyed in an incinerator. Psychiatrists attend training days, like the one Dr Tuke is at now, learning how to 'demonstrate' or 'show' empathy, as though we're at drama school. But we're never encouraged to genuinely try and put ourselves in our patients' hospital slippers. And to try and understand the cost-benefit analysis patients perform when they inevitably flush our medicines down the toilet.*

The pandemic has highlighted our ability to devise effective treatments rapidly, when we want to. But schizophrenia doesn't seem a priority for Big Pharma, or for society generally. You never see high-street charity chuggers collecting for 'schizophrenia research'. There have been no new breakthroughs in decades. No cleaner drugs have emerged. Just old formulas rebranded as new ones. And what has been invested is yet to bear fruit. The former head of the US National Institute of Mental Health admitted that during his tenure, despite NIMH throwing $20 billion at research into mental illness, it had failed to actually improve patients' lives.[1]

Consequently progress is slow, with patients lingering in hospital for months, years or decades. The 'get well soon' cards sold in the hospital gift shop seem gut-wrenchingly optimistic. On Friday mornings, when Dr Tuke is here, the PICU team are

---

* In the 1960s experimental psychiatrists not only sampled their patients' medicines but even sought to try and experience the symptoms of schizophrenia, albeit it transiently, by taking psychedelics to simulate the classic auditory and visual hallucinations. That was the justification for dropping acid on a workday, anyway, and spending twelve hours transfixed by the waves and folds of their corduroy trousers.

invited to share 'good-news stories'. Usually after an awkward silence my endlessly cheery Yorkshire consultant will say, 'Right, well have a good day everyone!' Recently our occupational therapist shared that a thirtysomething ex-mechanic had gone to the shops to buy some milk which was celebrated as though he'd scaled Mount Kilimanjaro.

'I don't *need* meds anyway,' Femi says. Whilst he no longer openly thinks he's a werewolf, he clearly still needs to develop better insight into his illness.

'Femi we're going to have to finish for now as I've got other patients to see. Have a think and let's come back to this later shall we?' I say, hoping a shiny, modern antipsychotic with no side effects and that definitely won't kill him might become available by the end of the day.

As I turn, my keys jangle on my belt buckle. Femi looks at them for a split second too long, so I start exiting the room.

'Femi you're doing really well so don't mess up your discharge, OK? I'll print you some information and see which medicine you'd mind the least. If you carry on like this, and we can switch your meds over, I think you'll be out in a week or two.'

After lunch Femi sees me talking to Reggie in the corridor and bounds over to us. I ready my well-worn explanation for why he still needs to take medicine and to stay in hospital a while longer.

'Doc I was thinking it'd be good to have a table-tennis tournament,' he says. 'Get everyone exercising.'

'That's a great idea Femi!' It's moments like this, seeing people get better, that make the job worth it.

'But it's too hot inside,' he adds, 'so let's do it in the garden.'

The 'garden' is the small outdoor concrete enclosure with an artificial grass lawn surrounded by an eighteen-foot-high perimeter fence.

Reggie looks to me. 'We're not really meant to take things out there.'

This is classic NHS bureaucratic bullshit. It's the same corporate, health-and-safety nonsense that disapproved of my 'bin lunches' on Daffodil Ward. Droplets of sweat are collecting on Femi's forehead.

He and most of the patients are in vests or topless and the temperature in here is bloody ridiculous. Plus the power I have over other people's basic human rights still doesn't sit easily with me. I want to embrace any compromises which might flatten the hierarchy.

'Reggie it's just a game of ping-pong!' I say.

'OK, but it's on you,' Reggie says.

Femi gives us both an elbow bump of appreciation and Reggie and I wheel the table-tennis table outside where the sun beats down on us.

'Maybe put it by the fence. So it's in the shade,' Femi suggests. He is full of good ideas today. Reggie and I do as we're told. Next the patients start heaving out the lead-weighted stools from inside for spectators to sit on.

Reggie looks to me again. 'We're not really supposed to—'

But I dismiss him. It's refreshing to see Femi and the others so empowered. They've slightly overdone it, bringing ten stools in total, but I don't want to be critical. And what could go wrong anyway?

'You wanna play bro?' Femi says, handing a paddle to a fellow patient called Emmanuel.

Others wander outside to watch, some of whom never usually get involved. We all become mesmerised by the satisfying rhythm of the game: *plink . . . pdonk . . . plink . . . pdonk*. Soon all the stools are taken.

Reggie and I look on proudly, happy to be included in the

patients' jokes and conversations. The boundaries between us dissolve and it briefly feels like there's no 'them' and 'us'. We could pass for a bunch of men at a park's outdoor table-tennis table on a summer morning.

'I need to start prepping afternoon meds,' Reggie says after a while, 'you OK to keep an eye on things here Benjamin?'

I nod and Reggie heads inside. Inevitably, several minutes later, my bleep sounds – I have to take a phone call. I look around for someone to cover, but we're short-staffed. The game continues being played in good spirits and I can't remember such a sense of harmony before. 'Just keep doing what you're doing, I'll be back in a minute,' I say.

I pop inside still smiling. We're now seeing the 'well' Femi; creative, friendly, looking out for everyone's physical wellbeing. He's not desperate to leave and seems to be gaining insight that for now hospital is the right place for him.

I answer my bleep; it's Dr Tuke just checking in and I tell him I've got everything under control. I hang up and follow the sound of whooping and cheering back into the garden. I *knew* outdoor ping-pong was a good idea!

On re-entering the garden I'm surprised to discover that the game has stopped. Instead, now on the table are *all* the lead-weighted stools, assorted like children's building blocks with Femi at the top of the precarious tower, looking up to the lip of the high fence.

'Femi stop! Come down!' I shout but I can't deny that the cheering is intoxicating. It's a thrilling moment: for Femi, the patients, and strangely even for me. In a split second I take it all in: the unity, the happiness, the awfully constructed tower Femi stands on top of. I'm horrified and impressed in equal measure. Was this a spur-of-the-moment job in Dr Tuke's absence, or a co-ordinated breakout attempt months in the making?

It's now or never to complete his great escape. If Femi can just make this jump he'll be a free man. He bends his knees, and pushes down hard. But it's a force too much for the flimsy table which buckles under its heavy load, and the stools, along with Femi, come crashing down.

The crowd groans in disappointment.

Hearing the bang, Reggie rushes outside. After shooting me a not subtle 'told you so' look, we help Femi hop to the clinical room, and as I'm bandaging his swollen ankle, applying some ice and ordering an X-ray, I think to myself that maybe some rules aren't totally ridiculous.

Later that afternoon Femi is a hero with the other patients. His exploits are legendary. During art group someone even reconstructs the scene as a painting, with the tower drawn almost as tall and just about as straight as that one in Pisa.

Among Reggie and other staff, I am simply the reason that the table-tennis table legs need replacing.

Now ping-pong is indoors again.

At the end of the day, I find Femi in the television room, where the patients are watching *Escape to the Country*.

If your ideal getaway involves an island retreat, why not consider Scotland's Outer Hebrides?

He gets up and hobbles over on his crutches. Luckily it was just a sprain. The corridor is largely empty except for Emmanuel loitering by the door, trying to 'act normal' on the off-chance that some naive agency worker who doesn't yet know the patients from the staff, will accidentally let him out. A less cinematic but far more common breakout method.*

---

* Unlike general nurses who wear an iconic light blue uniform, psychiatric nurses wear civilian clothes just like the patients. It's to reduce any sense of hierarchy but it does mean that the sane and the less sane look remarkably similar.

As we stand in the hot, claustrophobic corridors, illuminated by bright artificial lights, the TV continues burbling away, the happy couple talking . . .

We just felt so trapped living in the city. Now we're living the dream!

'Femi have you had a chance to read that information?'

'I'll just stick with the breast-milk meds for now,' he says. 'I guess it'll save me money on groceries.'

I smile. 'You'll be out of here soon then. But please just don't try anything like that over the weekend.' There are always even fewer staff at weekends, but I'd better not tell Femi that.

He smiles sheepishly. 'Sorry Doc.'

'How is your ankle anyway?'

'Sore. But it's OK. You alright?'

'Yeah, apart from you nearly giving me a heart attack,' I say and we laugh together.

I do feel OK. I'm surprised that my return to work hasn't been rockier. I seem to be in that proportion of people for whom the pandemic has brought either no change or even some improvement to their mental health. I'm grateful for the government-stamped excuse to retreat from modern life and to slow down. To press pause on a life lived in fast-forward. To not feel guilty about only leaving our flat for work. I'm also now making use of my daily allowance of exercise, and the more I run, the further I seem to leave the depression or whatever it is behind. Plus, our flat is calmer and my sleep has improved since only 'essential' businesses are open, which thankfully (at least for us) doesn't include bodybuilding gyms.

In the background an alarm sounds, and there's a brief panic as staff rush around looking for the source, then relax on discovering that it's coming from another ward. Then it stops.

It's the peaceful solitude that Nigel and Sheila love here by the sea!

Things have been progressing well with Esther too, besides the usual ups and downs. And this weekend we're 'taking the plunge', to use the property programmes' lingo, and moving in together: a tiny 'cottage' in London, which isn't silly rent, quiet, and even has a beautiful shared communal area at the back which I'm still excited about, despite today's experience of shared gardens.

Any end-of-the-week buoyancy in the staff certainly isn't shared by the patients, though. Despite the occasional drama, the more common complaint is the lack of things going on, as boredom sets in over the weeks, months or even years that patients stay here. Many no longer count the days, and the giant clock face on the front of the hospital has long stopped, to complete the feeling of time stood still.

On the TV the presenter continues wittering on.

Out here in the Hebrides there's just so much to do: hiking, swimming, stargazing or visiting one of the award-winning pubs . . .

'Could I get some leave over the weekend?' Femi asks.

'I don't think that's a good idea just yet,' I say. A common breakout method is for sectioned patients to persuade their psychiatrist to let them go for a walk or go to the shops as part of their rehabilitation. And then they'll bolt.* 'Let's discuss that next week,' I say.

---

* When patients abscond police are asked to return these AWOL patients to the ward. The trick here is not to go to the address on your NHS patient record. Many a patient has cracked open a celebratory beer in front of their TV, just as the flashing blue lights appear through their windows. Some craftier patients go further afield. I once phoned a patient who hadn't returned from his agreed six hours of leave and I was surprised to hear an international ringtone. 'So long, Dr Wankerhouse!' he said before putting the phone down, now safe on the beaches of Lisbon.

Femi nods wearily. 'You doing anything nice this bank holiday weekend Doc?'

Lockdown rules have eased further and the forecast is for clear blue skies over the coming days. Tomorrow I'm helping Sam move up to Sheffield where he has some silversmith friends and can afford the luxury of his own bedroom. On Sunday Esther and I are moving into our new rental, and on bank holiday Monday we're going for a socially distanced picnic in the park with Nafisa and her fiancé.

'Nothing much,' I say.

28

FAMILY

'Hello? Joseph can you hear me? I think you're on mute. That's it. Hang on, I'll just go somewhere more private,' I say, clutching my phone.

Esther has been furloughed by the temporarily closed Science Museum, so I shuffle past her in the living room and shut the bedroom door behind me.

'That's better,' I say, lying down on our bed.

The only catch with our own new 'space' is the lack of it. At just 400 square feet, the size of a two-car garage, the presenters on TV property programmes would creatively describe it as 'cosy'. Because there's only a shower, so I can continue my Radox therapy Esther got a bathtub off Gumtree and put it in the communal courtyard by our back door which at night I can fill with a hosepipe from the kitchen tap and cordon off with a shower curtain.

'So how're you both settling in?' Joseph asks.

I tell him that Esther and I are still getting used to living together. Small domestic things like our bedtime routine. To combat insomnia, after my bath I'll avoid caffeine and screens and wind down by reading medical journals in bed. Esther will hop in, we'll kiss goodnight and now drowsy we'll put the light out. A few minutes later Esther will turn it on again and say relaxing things like, 'We've not got enough money to make it through the month.' Then she'll switch it off again and say, 'Goodnight!'

Joseph laughs. 'As the saying goes, a problem shared is a problem handed over entirely to the other person.'

'Ha, yeah I suppose. We haven't killed each other yet, so that's good. Although . . .'

I tell Joseph about a fight I've just had with Esther about which way up I put cutlery in our drying rack. We moved in to develop a deeper understanding of one another and we're starting with washing-up preferences; she likes to put the blades up, whereas I put them down. I'm retelling my side of the argument when through the thin walls from the living room I hear . . . 'IT WASN'T LIKE THAT!'

I decide to finish my session in the park.

The Oedipus complex, as Joseph has frequently reminded me, is Freud's theory that romantically, boys unconsciously want to be with women like their mothers. I've always considered this fairly woo-woo since any women I'm attracted to are the exact opposite of my mother. My mum is white, fair-haired, fiery and very up-and-down. Whereas Esther is Southeast Asian, dark-haired, fiery and very up-and-down.

Often my mum would rationalise that the violence which happened under our roof, or sometimes spilled outside on to the bridge or in the barn, was mere evidence of love. 'We only fight because we care,' she'd tell me. 'If we didn't care we wouldn't bother fighting, would we?'

It's a warped logic but one I now subscribe to, that the intensity of feeling, of whatever sort, is synonymous with the strength of affection. It means that on the few occasions I dated calm, straightforward, well-adjusted women who wouldn't scream or shout, occasionally lash out or throw kettles of boiling water around, it just didn't feel right.

Esther, just like my mum, is a fighter, and I can accommodate that jagged jigsaw piece more naturally. The scary thing is that even if intellectually I sometimes query the wisdom of our relationship, I can't seem to stop my feet moving towards it.

'You find volatility familiar but at least you're working on yourself,' says Joseph. I'm now in the park sitting on a swing, an apt metaphor for the moods of the two most important women in my life. I'm a few hundred yards from our house and *hopefully* out of earshot of Esther.

Joseph has voiced concern that I may play out my parents' past mistakes with her, 'repetition compulsion' he calls it, but he says it doesn't have to be that way.

'Have you spoken to Esther yet about her getting some help?' he asks me.

'She says she can't afford it but it's her birthday next week so I've bought her some sessions as a gift.'

'Good present.'

'Inside her card I've written "Love you just the way you are, but . . ."'

Joseph laughs.

I don't think I'd be the first person to try and mould a partner to their liking. Even Henry VIII's sixth wife Catherine Parr must've looked at Henry's track record of two annulments, two executions and a death and still thought 'I can change him.'

'But generally things have been good,' I say. 'I sense we probably don't look dissimilar to those happy, normal-enough couples I used to envy. Just those little domestic things, you know?'

I tell Joseph that I no longer go to the supermarket alone. Now I go with Esther, who casually tosses things into the basket I'm carrying. Tyrrell's crisps and frozen chips mainly.

'I love that she doesn't even ask because now it's *our* basket.'

Almost miraculously, still no patients or relatives have tried to sue me, so each year my medical-insurance company continue issuing my £10 book voucher. The most recent addition to the bookshelf in my office is the self-help classic *The Road Less Travelled* by the psychiatrist Scott Peck.

Pre-COVID its wisdoms might have seemed trite, the sort of mush printed on tea towels. For example, on forgiveness Peck says there are personal benefits to forgiveness, since holding on to anger stops a person from growing. But during a global pandemic such messages have an increased resonance. Having the daily death tolls read out on the news before the football scores also highlights the fragility of life. It brings into focus not only what, but who, really matters. And if that wasn't enough of a push, today it's Father's Day.

I call our home landline and my dad answers. 'Hi Benji, sorry your mum's at the office,' he says. It's a Sunday but that doesn't always stop my mum from working.

'It's OK Dad, I actually wanted to talk to you.'

'Oh, that's nice.'

'Happy Father's Day too by the way.'

'Thanks love. And for the card.'

In WHSmiths the options for Father's Day cards all seemed to have illustrations of sheds on them, if not quite barns. The Mother's Day ones all bore glasses of white wine or gin and I wondered if maybe my parents aren't so different to everyone else's.

'That's OK Dad. How're you holding up? Are you getting a bit more energy?'

Despite living in the middle of nowhere, somehow my dad recently contracted coronavirus which hit him especially badly, and triggered a resurgence of his type II diabetes. 'I'm getting there. Feeling a bit stronger each day,' he says.

'Oh that's good. Well since it's Father's Day I just wanted to say . . .' I hover over my next sentence, something I can't remember saying to my dad before. My gut instinct is to mumble the

words, hide them under a cough or say them quickly. Instead, I
steady myself and take a breath. '. . . I just wanted to say, I love
you Dad. I'm sorry I never really say it.'

'Oh love, I love you too.'

My family have always been good at using terms of endear-
ment in place of our names, even during shouting matches. My
parents would scream at each other, 'I wish I'd never met you
darling!' or 'You ruined our fucking lives sweetheart!' The love
was never far away from the hate.

'Also Dad, I wanted to apologise. Growing up I think I told
myself you were a bad dad because of some of the things you did
to Mum and us boys, which neglected all the overwhelmingly
good things. So, I'm sorry about that.'

There's a pause. Nothing comes down the line for a moment.
Finally, my dad says, 'I often worried about how me and your
mum's behaviour would affect you boys growing up.'

With this sentence, one I will always remember verbatim, my
eyes glisten with tears which I intuitively push straight back. I
feel as though the heavy rucksack of family baggage I've been
lugging around, unsure if it was real or imagined or even mine
to carry, has been flung to the ground. I instantly feel lighter by
this admission from my dad. And that he even wondered about
the messy psychological shrapnel too.

And it was so effortless. It's like I've discovered a magic trick or
unlocked a 'cheat' to a computer game. My previous technique
of trying to force remorse from my parents only made them bris-
tle with defensiveness. But this way, by acknowledging my own
minor wrongdoing, my dad seems willing to follow my lead. It's
like I'm creating the space for an apology to fit into.

It's a rare departure from the party line that I had an 'idyllic
childhood', or being told that my worst memories were the
product of my imagination. This comment from my dad marks

a shift. As I once told Joseph, I never really cry, although no doubt that will catch up with me. It has with my dad and beneath his hardened skin is a kind and sensitive soul who now cries every few hours. I used to find it embarrassing but now it's just as regular as mealtimes.

The source of his tears is always a mystery. He'll cry during seemingly innocuous conversations, board games or a skilfully crafted pocket watch on the *Antiques Road Show*.

He was the firstborn of parents who had survived the Second World War, a no-nonsense, pull-your-socks-up generation who saw no reason for sorrow if you had carbohydrates, a roof and weren't being bombed. After a lifetime of repressed pain and a 'boys don't cry' philosophy, the ducts where tears are stored in my dad are so full, that the slightest flicker of emotion now causes their banks to overflow.

The tears aren't really for a valuable heirloom found in someone's loft, they're old tears from other times. I wish I could carbon-date them, as archaeologists can do with their ancient finds, to trace back their origins. My dad's had his fair share of trauma, sadness, disappointment and rejection. But I suspect a lot of his tears stem from regret about some of his previous actions.

'Thanks Dad, that really means a lot. Send my love to Mum and tell her I'll call next week.'

With this current window of openness, maybe I'll raise the topic with my mum again. It probably won't be any different from the hundreds of other times I've tried, but you never know.

After a stretch of night shifts, and COVID restrictions easing further, I have several days off, so with family on my mind I've decided to go and see my granny.

'Have you remembered I'm visiting you today?' I say on the phone that morning.

'Of course!' my granny fibs down the line. 'Let me just check I'm not doing anything.' I hear her good hand scrambling around for her paper diary on the laden trolley that contains everything she needs: the phone holster, her glasses, a hairbrush, the TV guide and a hundred biros that don't work. I'm not sure her diary is even this year's edition, but it hardly matters.

'I'm free!' she eventually says, and I can imagine her arthritic finger pressing down on the empty rectangle for today, surrounded by a sea of other white spaces.

Outside her front door I do a lateral flow which is negative. She's already had COVID anyway and brushed it off like the sniffles. Her back door is open as always. Inside I wash my hands and catch up with her carer Rita who is preparing lunch. I find my granny in her wheelchair in her usual place in the living room and plant a kiss on her cheek. People understandably keep their distance these days and she smiles at the physical touch.

'It's Benji here,' I tell her, taking her hand with a freshly alcohol-gelled one of my own.

'Oh, hello Benji!'

'Granny in future you should probably find out who the unknown, bearded men are *before* you let them kiss you.'

'You are good coming to see your silly old grandmother.'

'Not at all. Are you behaving?' I ask.

'Just about.'

Fighting fit into her nineties despite having not walked for fifteen years, she continues to defy medical science. My grandmother is indestructible.

'In case there's another lockdown I've brought you an early Christmas card and some flowers.'

'Oh they're beautiful. What are they?' She studies the yellow flowers on their long green stems as though trying to interpret hieroglyphics.

'They're tulips.'

'Oh yes,' she says.

I turn to greet the other person in her living room, sitting in his usual chair by the window.

'Hi Thomas,' I say to my uncle.

'Hello Benjamin,' he says in his usual monotone voice and we both exchange festive, red envelopes.

'How are you?' I ask breezily, trying to sound more like a nephew than a psychiatrist.

'I'm OK, yes I'm OK.'

'Well it's good to see you out of hospital.'

His eyes aren't wide and wild anymore. His bald head, a family trait, is leant back and he's rolling his neck around and around which is reassuringly 'Thomas-like'.

He was nearly right about the world ending. A global pandemic did wipe out millions. And now the climate crisis is causing biblical weather events, broadcast on the news almost daily. Not that Thomas is a modern-day Nostradamus, it was just an unhappy accident. Just as the broken clock on the front of the psychiatric hospital is right twice a day.

'It's a Friday which must mean we're getting a performance?' I say.

'That's right,' Thomas says sheepishly.

'Great I'll fix the teas,' I say.

I come back through from the kitchen with a tray of mugs and hold one to my grandmother's lips. One reliable constant is her unquenchable thirst for a brew.

Meanwhile Thomas has assembled his clarinet and is blowing air into the reed, causing startling noises to escape from the instrument.

'I'm just warming up,' he reassures us.

He recently started learning the clarinet and every Friday he comes and plays to my granny, which is ingenious because his paralysed, wheelchair-bound audience can't get away. He sometimes busks in the nearby town where he lives independently, and he's joked to me before that he's offered the most money to *stop* playing.

While my uncle is no Benny Goodman, he's undoubtedly a mental health success story. After his first admission aged twenty-four, he returned to employment, driving a van delivering parcels. He even later managed to return to his original job as an architect where, despite multiple relapses and hospitalisations, he worked for thirty years. Luckily by then he had a more understanding and supportive boss: my grandfather.

Thomas plays 'Greensleeves', 'Will Ye Go, Lassie, Go?' and 'We Wish You a Merry Christmas' with my granny singing along, the words still perfectly stored in some mysterious fold of her cerebrum. After thirty minutes he's puffed out and only half of his audience is still awake.

'All the excitement has tired Granny out,' I say, smiling at Thomas.

'She's OK. She's OK.'

'She is, yeah,' I say, knowing that's not quite the whole story.

Even when I'm with family I sometimes struggle to switch off the doctor part of me who is forced to give everyone I see a diagnosis. Be that asking Thomas (paranoid schizophrenia, F20.0) about his current antipsychotics, or informally monitoring the cognitive decline of my granny (vascular dementia, F01.0). I like to that think they're acts of love, a free medical consultation for my relatives without the wait.

'She is OK, but I think her dementia's getting worse, isn't it?' I add.

'Do you think?'

'Yep, 'fraid so.'

'I'm not sure,' my uncle says.

My granny's eyes open, maybe her ears burn or it's the smell of lunch wafting into the living room.

'Hello Granny, we were just talking about you,' I say.

'Oh dear, what have I done now?'

'Nothing, nothing,' I say stroking her arm. 'I was just wondering though, would you be up for playing a sort of game? It's just to test your memory.'

'Oh fine,' she says. 'No problems with my memory.'

I ask her the questions for an Abbreviated Mental Test Score, ten questions which screen for dementia. Questions like: where are we? What's your date of birth? And what are the dates of the Second World War?

'OK next question, who is the current prime minister?'

I think she might actually know this one, as her TV is always on and Boris Johnson is never out of the news.

'Oh yes, what's his name?' she says. 'That dishonest, bumbling Tory?'

I give her the mark for that.

Overall though, her low test score certainly screams of worsening dementia.

'And Granny, do you know who I am?' I point at my face to give her an extra clue. The test is over now. I just hate the idea of being a stranger to her.

She looks at me blankly.

'I'm Benji, your son John's eldest.'

'Oh Benji, hello dear,' she says. 'You are good coming to see your silly old grandmother.'

'I like coming. And who's this?' I point to Rita who's now entered with a water jug and some glasses. Rita is one of two

European carers who have helped cook for her, take her to the toilet, wash her and put her to bed for the last two decades. My granny looks at me bemused.

'Am I Filipa or am I *Rita*?' Rita says with emphasis.

'Filipa,' my granny says confidently.

'Nearly,' says Rita affectionately running her fingers through my granny's silver hair and returning to the kitchen.

I study my grandmother as she watches Thomas meticulously put away the individual pieces of his clarinet. For once the look on her face isn't one of confusion but lucidity and tender affection.

During my uncle's first long six-month psychiatric admission my grandmother dutifully visited Thomas second only to my dad. She always went alone, given my grandfather back then was one of those relatives who didn't or couldn't believe in mental illness. At least at the beginning.

But true love is unconditional, as my mum always reminded me in her own offbeat way. When tucking me into bed and saying she'd love me even if I went on a killing spree.

And it seems the feeling is mutual for Thomas and his mum. In the absence of a partner the main woman in his life is my granny, who he loyally visits three times a week.

On Tuesdays he does her shopping and odd jobs about the house. On Fridays Thomas plays her music. And at the weekend he wheels her to the church where for decades she ran the Sunday school, and afterwards they have lunch together.

He would admit to not being a natural conversationalist and they mostly just sit together. But it's a shared, loving silence and Thomas's quiet presence certainly doesn't go unnoticed.

'And who's this, Granny?' I say finally pointing to my uncle.

'That's Thomas,' she says without hesitation.

*

'Hello love, it's just me here,' my mum says on picking up the phone on Sunday. 'Dad's outside building the conservatory.'

'What do you mean "the conservatory"?'

'It's like a room with a glass roof and walls on the side of a house.'

I borrow a joke from *Fawlty Towers* that used to resonate with me and my brothers. 'Maybe afterwards he could move the house a bit to the left?'

'Ha ha,' she says sarcastically. 'It needed doing.'

'It's not exactly one of Maslow's Hierarchy of Needs is it Mum? Food, shelter, safety, summerhouse.'

'Maybe you'll understand if you ever own a house,' she says, and I laugh at the dig.

'Us boys can all support ourselves now so you could retire, Dad could stop building and you could actually start living your lives.'

'Please don't start that love. You say you can support yourselves but Sam's only just managed to get a bedroom for God's sake.'

I need to accept that my mum will always find something to worry about, and my dad will probably always try to stick extensions on to things. My dad's constant building is him striving towards a better life. And my mum's constant worry serves as a distraction from thinking about herself. But she never likes it when I put that to her.

'Chefs, artists and silversmiths don't exactly have much financial security,' she continues. 'At least I know you're alright because even NHS doctors in London can afford nice food and things.'

Now is *not* the time to tell her about my 'bin lunches' on Daffodil Ward.

'And all your cousins have children now too.'

About half of them do but my mum is no stranger to exaggeration.

'I would quite like to be a grandmother you know?' she continues. 'All I want is just one grandchild.'

I laugh hopelessly at the 'all I want' line. We've heard it so many times since that cameo-blue VW Beetle.

'Mum I'm sure one day one of us four will give you a grandchild. I actually wanted to speak to you about something else, if that's OK. You know how I've been having therapy?'

'Oh God, yes with that awful man Joseph. Is he making you think you had a terrible childhood again? I don't think he knows what he's talking about. Are you *sure* he's qualified?'

'Yeah Mum, he's qualified.'

'Well apart from helping with your dog phobia it sounds like he just stirs things up.'

'He just says that to move forward, you have to process the past. So I did just want to speak to you about a few things.'

'Uh oh,' my mum says, with nervous, pantomime dread.

The call with my dad was helpfully cathartic, so I'm just going to go for it.

'Mum it can't have been easy being the only woman at home. Whenever I tell people I have three brothers they always say, "Four boys? Your poor mum!" And it must've been really hard supporting the family financially with dad building the mill. I probably took that for granted so I'm sorry.'

'Thank you love.'

'And I know that often the simplest way to relieve that work stress, social isolation and the frustrations with dad was to pour a glass of—'

She coughs to interrupt me. 'Love can we do this tomorrow?' Her voice is panicky.

'Tomorrow?'

'Tomorrow yes, tomorrow. That would be better. Dad's not

come back in yet and we still need to have something to eat. Also I've got lots of ironing to—'

'It's just, that's what you said last time Mum.' I decide to plough on. 'I really just wanted to say I love you Mum and I'm sorry that I wasn't always able to protect you when things would kick off with Dad and . . .'

For some reason I'm crying now, which certainly wasn't in the script. I'm unable to finish my sentence and maybe this rare display of emotion is what tips my mum over the edge.

'Thank you for calling love but I just can't do this now, is that OK?' she says, her voice breaking, tears now free-flowing. 'I'm sorry I just can't do this now. I love you, darling. I love you so much,' she says, and then she puts down the phone.

29

NEW BEGINNINGS

After the country went into a last-minute, locked-down Christmas, it's New Year's Day and already 2021 is looking up. Today I'm getting vaccinated.

I walk through the hospital's automatic front doors where a thermal camera hanging from the ceiling shrieks in an automated voice 'Stop – high temperature detected!' The bored-looking NHS steward waves me in saying, 'They should never have put it by the entrance with an over-door heater.'

A woman with a 'volunteer' badge directs me to the makeshift vaccination hub, and following a straight, a left, a right, a straight, a lift down, then a left, a right and a left again, I am finally in completely the wrong place.

A whistling porter with a cage of laundry comes to my rescue. Porters are the endlessly cheery people who move things from ward to ward: bed linen, patients, cold bodies.

'Oh, you are lost,' he says when I tell him I'm looking for the vaccination hub. 'I'll take you. It's not very well signposted, to keep the anti-vaxxers out.'

But also the 'pro-vaxxers' it seems.

He drops me off there and when it's my turn, a nurse takes me into a small cubicle and I roll up my sleeve. 'So today we're giving you the Pfizer vaccine, it's one of the ones you've probably heard about,' she says. 'You wait ages for a vaccine and then three come along at once!'

One 'sharp scratch' later and I'm well on the way to coronavirus immunity. It feels so momentous and I thank her so profusely she says, 'You do know *I* didn't discover it?'

I know you didn't, I chased that guy down a street months ago!

I sit in a silent waiting room in case of an adverse reaction. It's a rare fifteen minutes of enforced reflection. The cure that everyone dreamed of is now a reality. The landmark vaccines have still come too late for millions around the world, though, including some front-line NHS workers and care staff. Like the lively receptionist with freckles in one of the A&Es I cover, who is now eerily absent.

Just as the creation of the NHS was the silver lining to the Second World War, surprisingly some good has sprouted from this crisis, the green shoots after a forest fire. With the planet on pause, wildlife is thriving and even in the city birdsong now wakes me and Esther each morning. The once-polluted canals of Venice are now said to be running clear. And reportedly the terror group ISIS has instructed its fighters not to target Europe for fear of infection. Every cloud.

I'm now in my final job of psychiatry training, which means in a year I'll be eligible to become a consultant.* A perk of being so senior is that my office in my new community job even has the luxury of natural light. My books on the shelf document my roller coaster of emotions over psychiatric training. My hardy, well-travelled cactus which has survived these years too, now sits on the sill, basking in the sunlight pouring through the window.

A recurring frustration of training is that I may only see a patient several times before moving on to a different placement. If I never see them again, I'm left to wonder how they are. Did

---

* Speciality training can be grim but thankfully, at least according to television, when I become a consultant someone from HR will give me an Aston Martin and some golf clubs.

they miraculously improve? Did they get worse? Are they still alive?

I'm left to ponder about the Malcolms who were socially distancing long before the pandemic started. The revolving-door Paiges bouncing in and out of hospital. The Sebastians for whom a chance encounter might offer another way out. The millions of Antons around the world who've been started on antidepressants since the pandemic began whose 'brain chemistry' seems to have mysteriously all dropped at exactly the same time.

Having now worked for many years in one NHS trust, covering the same geographical patch, I do occasionally come across old names and faces from previous placements or on-call shifts. It offers a rare glimpse of what traditional 'continuity of care' must have been like where some doctors knew their patients for a lifetime. It's dispiriting if I find such patients still as tormented as before. But it's not always like that.

A man my age, almost exactly my age, sits down. He's wearing clean clothes, a well-groomed beard. No rucksack or sleeping bag wrapped around his shoulders.

'Tariq it's good to see you again,' I say. 'I'm working in this team now. You look . . . different.'

Sometimes someone will survive a suicide attempt which defies the laws of science. A divine intervention or stroke of good fortune, depending on your parlance, will conspire to give a person a second chance in life. They will vomit up a deadly paracetamol overdose. They'll 'kick the bucket' and the rope or beam will snap instead of their neck. A hosepipe attached to an old exhaust will be looped through the car window, but then the engine won't start. Or as in Tariq's case, they'll fall fifteen metres from a bridge in pitch black and be cushioned by a deep thicket of brambles and shrubbery.

I last saw Tariq more than a year ago, on-call in A&E after he'd jumped. The dazzlingly lit A&E side room had contrasted so starkly with his bleakness. He hadn't had that regret that some survivors later describe the moment after their feet leave the metal railings of having made a terrible mistake. When the situation's gravity, in every sense of the word, hits them. Tariq had had no epiphanies, nor seen any white lights. His only regret had been that the attempt wasn't successful.

'How are you doing?' I ask.

'I'm OK. Good days and bad . . . mostly good now though.'

'And how was hospital?'

'It was alright, actually. Sorry about shouting at you that time in A&E, by the way.'

'That's alright. I don't imagine it's much fun being sectioned. Tell me what happened in hospital.'

'Well, I got that alcohol detox programme you were always banging on about. Got sober. I got involved in groups. Made a few friends there, ones who weren't pissheads. Social services managed to get me a house too. I mean, it is above an off-licence . . .' he adds with a wry smile.

I laugh, half in disbelief, and half not surprised at all.

'And the ward psychologist told me I needed to grieve or whatever . . . not just for Tyson, but for everything, you know?'

'I'm really sorry about Tyson.'

It feels strange seeing this smarter Tariq, in a different clinic room and without a perceived threat to my life, carpet or computer cables.

'He was old and I think I gave him an alright life.'

'And it looks like you've got new responsibilities?' I say looking at the bulldog puppy yawning in his lap.

'This is Holyfield,' he says.

We both chuckle and I glimpse Tariq's full smile for the first time.

Our appointment is nearly up. Tariq isn't depressed. He didn't need medication in hospital, just not to drink three litres of whisky a day, to talk to a therapist, to trust services to get him off the streets and to find something else to live for.

'Well done Tariq, seriously. People say beating alcohol is harder than heroin. I'm so pleased for you.'

He beams again.

'That's not an invitation to take up heroin by the way,' I add and we laugh together.

A sad reality about NHS psychiatry is that when patients recover you must say goodbye to them to make room for the next person in need.

'You don't look like you really need to be in this depression clinic. From the notes it seems like the drug and alcohol team are supporting you well. Do you feel ready to be discharged?'

'Sure,' he says.

While it's not a life entirely turned around, it's certainly a step in the right direction. It would be premature to think that Tariq will walk off into the sunset and live happily ever after. Di-Clemente and Prochaska's 'Stages of Change Model' identified the six phases of any behavioural modification as: Pre-contemplation, Contemplation, Preparation, Action, Maintenance, and somewhat ominously for some ends with Relapse. Probably with a slightly increased likelihood if you live above an offie selling two-for-one bottles of White Lightning. But for now, I'll drink a sparkling apple juice to Tariq's achievement.

Later, the usual doubt will creep in when I start to wonder if Tariq seemed almost *too* well? And I worry whether his cheery mood was *definitely* attributable to recovery and not that I'd just caught him right in that sweet spot a few drinks in?

'Tariq is there anything else you'd like to discuss before we finish?' I ask now.

'No I think that's it,' he says. He scoops the furry ball that is Holyfield up under his arm, stands and moves towards the exit. Then he says, 'Oh, there is just one thing.'

Oh God.

Some patients, often men, will put off raising difficult topics with their doctors until the very last minute. That's if they even seek medical advice at all. So sometimes, after what seemed an innocuous consultation, they'll drop an absolute bombshell. The practice even has its own name: 'the doorknob phenomenon'. Something like, 'By the way I've got crushing left-sided chest pain,' or 'What's the quickest way back to suicide bridge?' or 'Oh just one more thing, how can I get a Class 3 firearms licence?'

'What is it?' I ask.

'Oh, I err – just wanted to, say, you know . . .'

He holds eye contact with me before speaking, his once jaundiced yellow eyes now restored to a healthy cream colour.

'Thank you,' he says.

In this moment I think I understand Joseph's starfish fable and I blink back the water collecting in my eyes. Then I glance at my computer as though an email has caught my attention, as teary psychiatrists aren't really setting a good example in depression clinics.

But perhaps I should be pleased that I'm connecting, or maybe reconnecting, with my feelings after a horrible period of numbness. Earlier in my training I used to worry about my patients affecting me, but now I realise the far bigger problem is when compassion-fatigued psychiatrists get to the point that they don't.

I turn back to him. 'You're very welcome Tariq.'

'In case we never see each other again, would you like to stroke Holyfield before I go?' Tariq offers. 'It might be good for you.'

*

Before our first in-person therapy session in years, I use Joseph's new toilet.

He warned me during our Zooms that he'd spent lockdown redoing the bathroom. He said he was only telling me because the consistency of the therapeutic 'space' provides vital stability, and that previously people have broken down for as little as him hanging a new painting. I also sense part of him just wanted to show off the DIY handiwork of his lockdown project. So the 1970s avocado bathroom is out, and a new minimalist one is in. As I wash my hands in the angular sink, I think it's probably not the only thing that's changed.

When Joseph collects me for the first time in eighteen months, we meet each other's eyes and just about manage to hide our shock at how we've aged. Up close his hair is now entirely white, my first greys and early crow's feet wrinkles appearing.

'Hi!' he says warmly.

I automatically fall on to his familiar lumpy couch, the one I was so scared to lie on at first but the contours of which my back now knows. That spider, or maybe his progeny, is still on the ceiling. My head is closest to Joseph, so he no doubt has a view of my increasingly smooth crown. It must look like a bird's-eye view of a desert island where the tide is increasingly going out. When it comes to my balding, as I've matured I've just come to accept that I probably need to invest in a hair transplant.

I tilt my head back to look at him, but just get a view up his nostrils.

'It's nice to see you again Joseph. In 3D I mean.'

'You too. People say doing therapy on Zoom is like having sex with a condom on, it's not quite the same.'

'Very Freudian,' I say, wondering how safe Joseph's sex is.

'So what's new? Did you manage to get up north in the end?'

Restrictions being lifted means that, like lots of people, finally Esther and I got to reunite with our families in person.

I tell Joseph of how we'd got the train up to Newcastle together and didn't even have to hide in the toilets. Before entering the fusion restaurant to meet her mum and dad, Esther told me again that her Southeast Asian parents prefer talking about food to feelings. When I'd said I specialise in psychiatry her mum had smiled knowingly and said, 'So *that's* why you've ended up with Esther. She's the mad one in our family.' I'd asked Esther's mum if she was happy in her work and she'd waved her hands at me and said, 'No no no, I don't need therapy!' then she started recommending the dim sum. When the menu came Esther told them that I'd likely choose something bland because country people couldn't cope with spice. So I ordered something with three chilli logos besides it. The bubbling red curry was fine initially, but after thirty seconds I had to drink three glasses of water and a bowl of yoghurt.

I told Joseph that afterwards my dad had picked us both up and taken us to my family home in the middle of nowhere. And how Esther had said it was 'idyllic'.

'No, um, problems?' asks Joseph.

During lockdown Joseph would remind me that newspapers were reporting worrying spikes in domestic violence and home drinking. But the social isolation which I suspect partly drove this national trend, represented nothing new for my parents and they rode it out uneventfully.

'No, my parents are getting on pretty well these days actually.'

Time has softened the edges of my mum's anger and taken some of the intensity out of her emotions and reactivity. And now she just drinks at weekends. My dad is slowing down himself and becoming weaker, in town strangers sometimes offer to help carry his shopping bags. I haven't seen him lose his temper or be aggressive in years.

'Some things never change though,' I continue. 'My mum keeps taking on new cases, even though she's supposedly retiring. I'm starting to think she'd be more stressed if she wasn't working.' Joseph smiles in recognition. He must now be pushing seventy himself. 'And my dad keeps tweaking our house, moving rooms around. I went to use the downstairs toilet and for some reason he's turned it into a mini second kitchen.'

Joseph laughs. 'Your mother needs to keep up her professional walls, and your father needs to keep building actual ones.' Despite his age, Joseph's still got it. 'What did your family make of Esther?'

'I think they liked her. They say she's funny. But intense.'

'You like intense,' Joseph says and we both laugh.

'And my mum didn't even tell me to break up with her, which is progress. And soon there'll be one more of us at our family gatherings,' I continue excitedly.

As I've grown up, my family have always quietly, and not-so-quietly in my mum's and grandmothers' cases, wondered why my brothers and I are so far behind our cousins in establishing relationships and having kids. Beyond the small biological hurdle of me not previously having had a serious partner, I've sometimes worried if I'd be a bad dad or rear unhappy offspring. But my brother Josh is throwing caution to the wind.

Several weeks ago on Christmas Day during lockdown, my family opened their Secret Santa gifts on Zoom from their respective homes. Josh gifted my mum a book called *The Good Granny Guide*. When the penny eventually dropped (helped by the baby ultrasound scan inside) my mum jumped up, hugged my dad and ran around the kitchen with happiness.

'They're having a boy,' I continue. 'Our family only knows how to make boys.'

Ahead of our visit my mum had got all our old children's clothes down from the loft to pass on to Finan when he's born. Blue and white striped dungarees and handmade patchwork quilts, perfectly preserved. And my dad dug out old camcorder footage that he'd taken of us boys doing funny things as babies, and when we watched them – true to form – he cried throughout.

Because if there is a gene lurking somewhere in my family's DNA for schizophrenia, violence, alcoholism or male-pattern balding, there is also undeniably one for love.

'My parents are good people, you know Joseph.'

'I know,' he says sincerely.

We sit for a minute in contemplative silence until Joseph is unable to hold it in any longer.

'So what do you think of my new bathroom?' he says.

ACKNOWLEDGEMENTS

Firstly, thank you to my family for letting me tell our story, or at least my version of things.

To my three not-so-little brothers Josh, Gabe and Sam for the endless phone calls corroborating real and misremembered memories.

To my mum and dad for coming round to this quite modern idea of talking about difficult things, instead of ignoring them and hoping they'll go away. And for letting me write chunks of this in our caravan at the end of the field. Turns out sometimes complete isolation can be a good thing. I love you both.

To my wise and diligent agent Lucy Morris at Curtis Brown, force of nature Cathryn Summerhayes who first took a punt on me, and to super-sub Rosie Pierce.

To Curtis Brown Creative, the online writing course I did in lockdown, tutored by the excellent Cathy Rentzenbrink. And to Jennifer Kerslake who offered to send my writing to agents and got me one within the hour.

To the publishing team at Jonathan Cape and Vintage. Specifically to my editors Bea Hemming and Jenny Dean for their endless calm and enthusiasm respectively. You perhaps now regret telling me that some authors submit manuscripts ten years late. So my two years isn't so bad.

Special thanks to Jamie Coleman who came in late and is nothing short of a book wizard.

To copy-editor David Milner for tolerating my never-ending changes.

And to the publicity, marketing and sales teams at Vintage:

Mia Quibell-Smith, Maya Koffi, Katrina Northern and Amelia Rushen for promoting my book.

To Esther, who is so many people's favourite character, in the book and in real life.

To my 'granny' who is really an amalgam of both my amazing grandmothers.

To my uncle for his blessing to be included too.

To my therapist Joseph, obviously.

Thanks to those comedian friends who offered their thoughts: Jake Baker, Rich Hardisty, Matt Hutchinson, Ed Patrick, Johnny White Really-Really, Ian Smith, Dave Green, Ben Clover and Jordan Brookes. Richard Todd especially helped me to squeeze more out of scenes. Dan Audritt and Kat Butterfield can see the funny in anything, and Chris Stokes came up with the title. There are others too but I'm already over my word count, you know who you are.

To my oldest pals Al, Henry, Nafisa, Si, Matty, Bas, Felix, Ol, Pete, Nick, Dragon and Jenny for their phone calls, encouragement and for coming to chapter read-throughs.

To The Moth, the international storytelling institution where as host of the London night I learnt how to tell real-life five-minute stories before moving on to the more daunting task of writing an 80,000-word one.

To the endlessly patient Juliette, Harriet, Molly and Cal at House Productions for imagining my book on the screen. And to Susanna Waters, who I met on the CBC screenwriting course, for her helpful input.

To the makers of Jaffa Cakes and Yorkshire Tea for keeping me nourished and focused during the writing process. I couldn't have done it without you.

To the psychiatry friends who read early drafts and offered guidance on how not to get struck off: Max Pemberton, Amy

Jebreel, Dan Hughes, Senem Leveson, Laura Korb, Jonny Martell, Mark Horowitz and Graham Campbell. To the historical psychiatrists, good and not-so-good, whose names I've borrowed for characters within the book. And to those colleagues who strive to make psychiatry more compassionate and humane in the future.

And finally, of course, thank you to my patients.

USEFUL NUMBERS

Samaritans is a confidential listening service available 24-hours a day, 365 days a year. 116 123.

Campaign Against Living Miserably (CALM) offer something similar 5 p.m. to midnight. 0800 585858.

Childline is available for those under nineteen. 0800 1111.

For those who prefer messaging, text 'SHOUT' to 85258.

Students can find university or college listening services on Nightline (www.nightline.ac.uk).

Switchboard are especially LGBTQ+ friendly. 0800 0119 100.

Refuge is a confidential 24-hour domestic abuse helpline. 0808 2000 247.

Mind is a mental health charity and an excellent general resource (www.mind.org.uk).

If it's an emergency, please call 999, your local crisis team, or attend A&E.

NOTES ON SOURCES

Preface

1 According to the Centre for Mental Health, accessed 2023. www.centrefor mentalhealth.org.uk/parity-esteem.

2 According to NHS England, accessed 2023. www.england.nhs.uk/statistics /statistical-work-areas/bed-availability-and-occupancy/bed-data-overnight/.

3 According to the Royal College of Psychiatrists, 2019. www.rcpsych.ac .uk/news-and-features/latest-news/detail/2019/11/05/hundreds-more -psychiatric-beds-needed-to-help-end-practice-of-sending-patients -hundreds-of-miles-for-treatment-says-rcpsych.

Chapter 1

1 According to the British Medical Association, 2023. www.bma.org.uk /bma-media-centre/junior-doctors-can-make-more-serving-coffee-than -saving-patients-bma-warns-ahead-of-three-day-strike.

Chapter 3

1 Andrew Scull, *Madness in Civilization* (Thames & Hudson, 2015).

Chapter 7

1 Aamna Mohdin, 'Mental Health Act reforms aim to tackle high rate of black people sectioned', *Guardian*, 13 January 2021.

Chapter 8

1 Peter Moszynski, 'GMC to look into higher number of complaints against overseas trained doctors', *British Medical Journal*, 1 August 2007.

Chapter 10

1 Luke Sheridan Rains et al., 'Understanding increasing rates of psychiatric

hospital detentions in England: development and preliminary testing of an explanatory model', *BJPsych Open*, 14 August 2020.

Chapter 20

1 National Confidential Inquiry into Suicide and Safety in Mental Health (NCISH), 2016.
2 'Homicide in England and Wales: year ending March 2022', Office for National Statistics, 2022.

Chapter 23

1 Joanna Moncrieff et al., 'The serotonin theory of depression: a systematic umbrella review of the evidence', *Molecular Psychiatry*, 20 July 2022.
2 C. M. France, P. H. Lysaker & R. P. Robinson, 'The "chemical imbalance" explanation for depression: Origins, lay endorsement, and clinical implications', *Professional Psychology: Research and Practice*, 38(4), 2007.
3 Andrea Cipriani et al., 'Comparative efficacy and acceptability of 21 antidepressant drugs for the acute treatment of adults with major depressive disorder: a systematic review and network meta-analysis', *Lancet*, 21 February 2018.
4 James Davies, *Sedated: How Modern Capitalism Created Our Mental Health Crisis* (Atlantic Books, 2022).

Chapter 26

1 Adam O. Horvath & B. Dianne Symonds, 'Relation between working alliance and outcome in psychotherapy: A meta-analysis', *Journal of Counseling Psychology* 38(2), 1991.

Chapter 27

1 Adam Rogers, 'Star Neuroscientist Tom Insel Leaves the Google-spawned Verily for . . . a Start-up?', *Wired*, 11 May 2017, www.wired.com/2017/05/star-neuroscientist-tom-insel-leaves-google-spawned-verily-startup/?mbid=social_twitter_onsiteshare.

ABOUT THE AUTHOR

Dr Benji Waterhouse is a front-line NHS doctor specialising in psychiatry. He is also an award-winning stand-up comedian who performs sell-out shows at the Edinburgh Festival. He has written for the *Guardian* and *Independent* and was included in a list of 'Inspiring Psychiatrists' by the Royal College of Psychiatrists. *You Don't Have to Be Mad to Work Here* is his first book.

linktr.ee/dr_benji
X doctor_benji
O doctor_benjis